Praise for *The Alzheimer's Prevention & Treatment Diet*

"Cutting-edge approach"

"Dr. Isaacson is a renowned expert who blends advanced science with practical insights for the new standard of treatment and prevention. His cutting-edge approach is exactly where we need to be in the fight against Alzheimer's disease."

–Dr. Arthur Agatston, MD, Cardiologist
New York Times best-selling author of *The South Beach Diet*™

"Empowering"

"A refreshingly optimistic perspective on prevention and treatment for a disease that has confronted many disappointed therapies. It is empowering for patients, caregivers, and clinicians."

–Dr. Daniel A. Cohen, MD, MMSc
Cognitive Neurologist, Eastern Virginia Medical School

"A valuable resource"

"*The Alzheimer's Prevention & Treatment Diet* is not only based on the most up-to-date knowledge and studies in the field, but also designed to be easily followed by anyone who's interested in maintaining and enhancing cognitive health. Here is a valuable resource that I can heartily recommend!"

–Dr. Dale V. Atkins, PhD, Psychologist
Author of *Sanity Savers*

"The perfect guide"

"Dr. Isaacson has devoted his career to fighting Alzheimer's. He's taught me that our diets play a major role in keeping our brains healthy. This book is the perfect guide for people who want to do just that."

–Dan Pashman
Host of the Cooking Channel series *You're Eating It Wrong*
and author of *Eat More Better*

———◆———

"It can work for you"

"*The Alzheimer's Prevention & Treatment Diet* will surprise you as it offers readers an ability to substantially improve brain health through nutrition. I personally know patients of Dr. Isaacson. This approach has worked for them and it can work for you."

–David Pottruck
New York Times best-selling author of *Clicks and Mortar*

———◆———

"Latest findings in the field"

"I would recommend anyone to follow closely the work of Dr. Isaacson and see him as a patient for prevention. He is a leader working to end the era of "diagnose and adios" for brain disease. This work presents the latest findings in the field matched with rigorous clinical validation."

–Max Lugavere, Filmmaker
Director and Producer of *Bread Head*

The
ALZHEIMER'S PREVENTION &TREATMENT

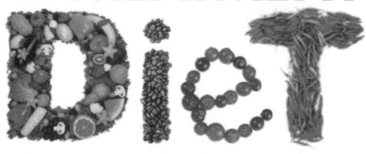

Diet

USING NUTRITION TO COMBAT THE EFFECTS OF ALZHEIMER'S DISEASE

RICHARD S. ISAACSON, MD
CHRISTOPHER N. OCHNER, PhD

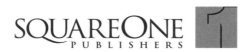

SQUAREONE
PUBLISHERS

The information and advice contained in this book are based upon the research and the professional experiences of the authors, and are not intended as a substitute for consulting with a healthcare professional. The publisher and authors are not responsible for any adverse effects or consequences resulting from the use of any of the suggestions discussed in this book. All matters pertaining to your physical health, including your diet, should be supervised by a healthcare professional who can provide medical care that is tailored to meet individual needs.

COVER DESIGNER: Jeannie Tudor
TYPESETTER: Gary A. Rosenberg
IN-HOUSE EDITOR: Joanne Abrams

Square One Publishers
115 Herricks Road
Garden City Park, NY 11040
(516) 535-2010 • (877) 900-BOOK • www.squareonepublishers.com

Library of Congress Cataloging-in-Publication Data
Names: Isaacson, Richard S., author. | Ochner, Christopher N., author. Title: The Alzheimer's prevention & treatment diet : using nutrition to combat the effects of Alzheimer's disease / Richard S. Isaacson, MD, Christopher N. Ochner, PhD.
Other titles: Alzheimer's prevention and treatment diet
Description: Garden City Park, NY : Square One Publishers, [2016] | Includes bibliographical references and index.
Identifiers: LCCN 2016005347 (print) | LCCN 2016005874 (ebook) | ISBN 9780757004087 (pbk.) | ISBN 9780757054082 (epub) | ISBN 9780757054082
Subjects: LCSH: Alzheimer's disease—Prevention—Popular works. | Alzheimer's disease—Diet therapy—Popular works.
Classification: LCC RC523.2 .I83 2016 (print) | LCC RC523.2 (ebook) | DDC 616.8/310654—dc23
LC record available at http://lccn.loc.gov/2016005347

Printed in the United States of America

10   9   8   7   6   5   4   3   2   1

Contents

To my patients and their family members,
who have committed themselves to the fight against Alzheimer's,
and taught me volumes in the process.
Your courage is inspiring to me every day.
And to Drs. Robert Krikorian and Sam Henderson,
pioneers in Alzheimer's nutrition research.

—RSI

To Ron and Mae,
the most supportive, caring, and loving parents
with whom anyone could be blessed.
Thank you.

—CNO

Acknowledgments

This book would not be possible without the help and collaboration of many individuals. A special thanks to my family, who have all played a significant role in my development as a person and as a physician. My dad was my biggest role model, and I would be remiss without thanking my mom for her love, resilience, and proofreading skills. I also thank my sister Suzee-Q, brother Stewie, brother in-law Mike, nieces, nephews, grand-niece Brielle, and cousin Stacy

I am grateful to my mentors, supervisors, and colleagues: Drs. Chris Papasian, Clifford Saper, Michael Ronthal, Louis Caplan, Ralph Sacco, Matt Fink, Laurie Glimcher, Joe Safdieh, Dan Cohen, Cindy Zadikoff, Sean Savitz, Michael Benatar, Ralph Józefowicz, Alon Seifan, and Ranee Niles.

I thank the Helfner family; all my teachers/advisors at Commack High School, including Jack McGrath, Ron Vale, Dr. Doug, and Susan Dreilinger; Christine Greer, Mimi, Grey, Rach, and Bon Bon; Liz Greer and Oma; Sara Fusco; my best friends, Dave Acevedo, Reza Khan, Brett Helfner, Chris Ochner, Justin Berger, Mike Haff, Harold Levy, Brandon Suedekum, Tonnie Markley, Janie Fossner-Pashman, Brian Martin, Wilfried Baudouin, Dr. Andy Tarulli, and H. Ron Davidson; Dr. Islon Woolf; and Dr. Dale Atkins.

A sincere thank-you to Suzanne Summer, MS, RD, for the development of sample menus and for her valuable insights and consultation on nutrition information provided in the chapter "The APT Diet." Thanks also go to Rudy Shur, Joanne Abrams, and Miye Bromberg of Square One Publishers; Carol and Gary Rosenberg; Max Lugavere; the APC team (Dr. Alon Seifan, Mary Montgomery, Roberta Marongiu, Dr. Randy Cohen, Jaclyn Chen, Katherine Hackett, Jeannette Hogg, Chefi Meléndez-Cabrero, and Cindy Shih); Ciara Gaglio, Mark McInnis, Genevieve LaBelle, Jason Goldstein, and the entire AlzU.org team; Christina Stolfo-Rupolo; Ashley Paskalis; Janice Void; Anthony Galindez; Lewis Cruz; Tom Horton; Dr. Greta Strong; Dr. Larry Newman; Mary Hopkins and Kathy Bradley from JHC; Dr. Edmond Mukamal; the Regenerates; the Principality of Monaco; and the New York Yankees.

—RSI

I would like to thank my parents who continue to inspire me. Your unconditional love and support made me everything I am today and will be tomorrow. Thank you for not only being the most amazing parents but also great editors. To Dr. Robert Scott Ochner, the only family member to escape having to read this book several times. I miss you, Bobby. To my brother Ricky and sister Cheryl, you have both been siblings, parents, and best friends to me. Thank you not only for helping with this book, but also for guiding me throughout my life.

To John Spychalski. You were one of the most influential components of my development, both personal and professional, and will always be a close friend. To Dr. Michael Lowe, for your mentorship, support, and friendship, and for proving that honesty and integrity are not preclusions to success. To Dr. Stephen Bono, for being a continual mentor and friend. Your support and guidance are never taken for granted.

To Dr. Eric Stice, for being a role model and demonstrating just how much one person can do and achieve while maintaining balance in life. To Dr. Xavier Pi-Sunyer, for your continued support and guidance.

To the Irving Institute for Clinical and Translational Research, the New York Obesity Nutrition Research Center, the Mount Sinai Adolescent Health Center, and the National Institutes of Health for supporting my research. To my outstanding graduate students from the Columbia University Institute of Human Nutrition for your help and future contributions as outstanding physicians.

To my coauthor, colleague, and friend, Dr. Richard Isaacson. After all the sleepless nights, "work retreats," and "spirited discussions," I am extremely proud of what we have accomplished. The different styles we brought to this process have culminated in something very special, and the ability to create resources for helping others with my close friend is truly a unique privilege.

Finally, to my loving wife, Angel. You inspire me to be a better person every day, and I will never stop appreciating that. Thank you for understanding when I couldn't be there and for always being there when I needed you. No matter what "it" is, I couldn't do it without you . . . and wouldn't want to. I love you.

—CNO

Preface

For years, patients, caregivers, family members, and clinicians have been actively searching for new approaches to managing Alzheimer's disease (AD). Recently, there has been an explosion in research on nutritional interventions for preventing and treating this disorder. While diet has historically been a critical component of the therapeutic plans for many other chronic diseases, including diabetes, high blood pressure, and high cholesterol, it's only in the last decade or two that scientists have begun to investigate the impact of diet on brain health. So far, the results have been promising. The latest studies offer new hope for people concerned about memory loss, presenting extensive scientific evidence that diet can be an effective tool for supporting and even improving cognition. Clearly, the tide has begun to turn toward the "brain-healthy diet" as an essential part of Alzheimer's disease management.

Dr. Isaacson is a neurologist who specializes in Alzheimer's disease; Dr. Ochner is a clinical scientist who focuses on nutrition. Our daily efforts concentrate on three areas: education, research, and patient care. We teach other physicians and researchers, as well as medical and graduate students, at large and well-respected academic medical centers in the United States. We work with doctors, scientists, psychologists, nurses, nurse practitioners, trainees, and other members of the healthcare team. We have published our research on

Alzheimer's disease in internationally recognized medical journals and presented our work throughout the world. And we have worked closely with patients—many of whom are in good cognitive health and want to avoid developing Alzheimer's, while others are in the early stages of Alzheimer's and hope to slow the disorder's progress. Through our work with virtually thousands of patients, we have come to recognize the need to not simply provide an optimal diet, but also help people understand the principles of brain-healthy nutrition; gradually transition from their present way of eating to a food plan that protects and enhances cognitive well-being; and incorporate other practices, such as exercise, to create a comprehensive brain-healthy lifestyle. *The Alzheimer's Prevention and Treatment Diet* is the culmination of our efforts.

This book is, first and foremost, based on studies which show that specific nutrients, foods, dietary patterns, and lifestyle practices can help protect brain health. But it is also based on our firsthand experience in working with patients over the long term. We have learned that if people are going to follow a diet not just for a few weeks but for the rest of their lives, it is necessary to create a plan that is satisfying to both the brain *and* the belly. Therefore, we have incorporated strategies and tactics that have proven successful in our practice. We are proud that our diet plan can be followed by real people living in the real world.

Despite the wealth of evidence supporting a role for diet in AD prevention and treatment, the benefits of nutrition are still not widely acknowledged. We hope that this book raises awareness of the importance of diet for optimal brain health. While you can't control every aspect of your health, there are many things that you can do to keep your mind sharp and agile and to improve the overall quality of your life. By adjusting your eating habits and making some simple lifestyle changes, you can have a positive impact on your brain and body for years to come.

Introduction

The Alzheimer's epidemic may be the greatest public health crisis facing our world today. There are over 5 million Americans with Alzheimer's disease (AD), and millions more are affected throughout Canada, Europe, Australia, and the rest of the world. One out of nine people age sixty-five and over has dementia, and over a third of individuals over the age of eighty-five have AD. The increasing prevalence of Alzheimer's disease is due in part to the advancing age of our population. Advancing age is the primary risk factor for AD, and with more and more baby boomers turning sixty-five every year, the number of AD cases is projected to more than triple by the year 2050!

But while advancing age may be the biggest factor behind the rise of Alzheimer's disease, it is not the sole factor. Poor dietary habits also play an important role. It turns out that the foods you eat have an enormous effect on your risk of Alzheimer's disease. An unhealthy diet not only contributes to obesity, diabetes, cardiovascular disease, and metabolic syndrome—all conditions that seem to increase the risk of dementia—but may also directly influence the ways in which your brain works. Poor lifestyle habits, such as a lack of exercise, are also associated with a higher risk of AD.

The good news is that diet and other lifestyle practices are well within your control. Based on the most recent scientific research, and supported by our real-life experience working with patients, *The Alzheimer's Prevention and Treatment Diet* will give you the dietary strategies you need to enhance your well-being, strengthen the health of your brain, and improve your ability to fight Alzheimer's disease. We've shared these strategies with our patients and our own family members, and now we'd like to share them with you. That's because anyone and everyone—be they twenty-nine or ninety years of age— can make the lifestyle changes that lead to better health and cognition. Our goal is to guide you in making choices that will not only improve your overall well-being but also protect your brain.

The first four chapters of *The Alzheimer's Prevention and Treatment Diet* offer the information you need to understand Alzheimer's, the link between Alzheimer's and nutrition, and our diet program. Chapter 1 presents a comprehensive overview of Alzheimer's disease, detailing AD's stages and symptoms, explaining the difference between age-related cognitive decline and cognitive decline due to AD, and looking at the condition's causes and risk factors. The chapter ends with a brief discussion of AD diagnosis and AD research trials.

Chapter 2 zeroes in on our focus of prevention through diet by answering the question, "Why does diet matter?" The chapter first looks at the various ways in which foods can affect the brain. It then examines two nutrition-related health problems—excess body fat and diabetes—and discusses their association with Alzheimer's disease. Finally, it introduces new dietary concepts that may hold the keys to the future of AD prevention and treatment.

The dietary strategies and guidelines that form the foundation of the Alzheimer's Prevention and Treatment Diet are based on the effect that the substances known as *macronutrients*—carbohydrates, protein, and fats—have on health in general and brain health in particular. Chapter 3 provides basic information about these dietary components and explains how by carefully selecting both the quantity and the quality of your carbs, proteins, and fats, you can help protect brain and memory function.

Over the last few decades, there has been increased interest in the use of nutrition to enhance brain health and avoid or manage neurological disorders such as AD. Studies have explored a range of specific nutrients, specific foods, dietary patterns, and other approaches that that may have the potential to prevent or treat cognitive decline. Chapter 4 focuses on the most important of these studies and diets, including the Mediterranean diet, the ketogenic diet, the MIND diet, calorie-restrictive diets, and the FINGER study. It then turns its attention to the Alzheimer's Prevention and Treatment Diet, which takes into consideration all of the latest evidence on AD—including the studies presented in the chapter—but integrates unique elements that contribute to its effectiveness and accessibility.

Chapters 5, 6, and 7 put the information from the earlier chapters into action by presenting a practical guide to making dietary and other lifestyle changes necessary to prevent, delay the onset, or slow the progression of Alzheimer's disease. Here, you'll find what you need to know to protect and enhance your cognitive health.

Chapter 5 is a step-by-step guide to our nine-week diet plan. The chapter begins by explaining the dietary goals of the Alzheimer's Prevention and Treatment Diet. Then, for each week, we instruct you in planning and preparing for that week's dietary and lifestyle changes; provide specific dietary guidelines; and recommend exercise and other activities that can further enhance your cognitive well-being. This proven approach gradually introduces change into your life and also enables you to successfully face any challenges you may encounter, from eating on the go to dining out. Lists of recommended foods and brain-healthy snacks, a special section on meal replacements, and sample menus ease your transition to a brain-healthy lifestyle.

Although diet is one of the most important weapons we have in the fight against Alzheimer's disease, it is not the only weapon. Research has shown that the best way to prevent and treat Alzheimer's is to use a multifaceted approach that includes specific nutritional supplements, physical exercise, stimulating intellectual and social activities, and stress-reduction techniques. Chapter 6 guides you in successfully using these approaches to not only protect your brain but also enhance the quality of your everyday life.

As the name suggests, the Alzheimer's Prevention and Treatment Diet is designed to both prevent the development of cognitive problems and slow further decline in those who have already been diagnosed with the disease. However, as AD progresses, it can become difficult to maintain optimum nutrition. Chapter 7 explores the problems that may develop with the onset of AD symptoms and offers proven tips for managing them so that the person with AD can receive the best nutrition possible. Since diet can be affected—for better or worse—by medication, this chapter also looks at the medications most often prescribed to manage the symptoms of AD and guides you in timing meals and drug therapy so that they work hand in hand. Finally, Chapter 7 provides helpful tips and strategies for caregivers and others who have people with AD in their life.

We have tried to make the information in this book easy to understand and to keep the use of medical- and nutrition-related terminology to a minimum. You will not need a medical degree to understand the science behind our diet program! But some terminology is necessary to explain brain function and the impact that foods and their nutrients have on the body. With this in mind, we created a Glossary (page 215) that defines the terms used in our book. Turn to it whenever you want to double-check the meaning of a word or phrase with which you're not familiar.

Throughout the book, we emphasize the importance of understanding AD as well as the effect that nutrition can have on your brain so that you can make the best dietary choices possible. This book provides a solid foundation of knowledge, but it's important that you have access to further information so that you can continue to follow a healthy diet throughout your life. That's why we have compiled a comprehensive Resources list, which not only guides you to websites that can offer detailed nutritional data, but also suggests organizations and sites that provide a wealth of information on Alzheimer's disease, its risk factors, its stages, its management, and other topics of interest. Also included are organizations geared to assist family members who serve as caregivers for people with AD.

Finally, we've given you log sheets to help you track your progress in adopting a brain-healthy diet. In these logs, you'll record food intake; jot down the carbohydrate counts that are so important to the APT Diet; and make lists of favorite foods, brain-healthy snacks, and more—all with the goal of helping you implement positive changes. If you prefer, you can track your progress online with the Alzheimer's Disease-Nutrition Tracking System (AD-NTS), which is available on the Alzheimer's Universe website. (See page 232 of the Resources list.)

Everybody has the potential to lead a brain-healthier life, and our gradual approach to dietary and lifestyle changes maximizes your chance of success. As you continue on the Alzheimer's Prevention and Treatment Diet, remember that Rome wasn't built in a day, and neither is a brain-protective lifestyle. Over time, the small changes that you begin implementing today will pay off. There is no more important investment than the investment you make in your health.

1.

Understanding
Alzheimer's Disease

Before we get into the details of the Alzheimer's Prevention and Treatment Diet, it's important that you know a little about the disease itself. Alzheimer's disease (AD) is a *neurodegenerative disease*—that is, a disease that causes the progressive destruction of neurons (brain cells). As the neurons die, the brain loses its capacity to function normally, resulting in a gradual decline in memory and other cognitive skills. Accordingly, Alzheimer's disease is the most common cause of dementia, accounting for at least two-thirds of all diagnosed cases.

Because AD is increasingly prevalent in the world today, many people are already somewhat familiar with it. The disease has several different stages and phases, each with its own specific challenges for caregivers, family members, and diagnosed individuals. Education is one of the best tools we have to fight Alzheimer's. By familiarizing yourself with the disease, you'll be taking the first step in learning how to best manage it.

This chapter will provide you with a comprehensive overview of Alzheimer's disease. Using the most current information, we detail the disease's symptoms and risk factors, outline its characteristic brain changes, and describe the diagnostic process and available management options. We also explain how Alzheimer's disease differs from normal age-associated cognitive decline. With this basic foundation of knowledge about AD, you'll be better equipped to understand why it is so important to take steps now to prevent or slow down the progression of this condition. And you'll have a far clearer sense of why our approach to Alzheimer's disease makes sense. Let's get started!

THE STAGES AND SYMPTOMS OF AD

When most people think about Alzheimer's disease, they associate it with forgetfulness or memory loss. But there are many other symptoms of Alzheimer's. Sometimes the first observable sign of AD is not

Dr. Isaacson's Uncle Bob, Age Twenty-Nine

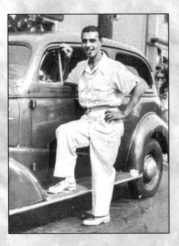

Here's my Great-Uncle Bob at the age of twenty-nine. Uncle Bob was especially important to me. Not only is he the reason I'm here today—he introduced my parents and saved my life when I was a toddler—but he sparked my interest in the field of Alzheimer's disease.

When I think of my Uncle Bob, the first words that come to mind are, "What a party!" Uncle Bob was always happy—smiling, telling jokes, the life of the party. He started having memory trouble in the early 1990s, back when I was in high school. He was formally diagnosed with AD just as I was finishing college and about to start medical school. As I continued my studies, I was frustrated to find that even though medicine had come such a long way, there were still no real treatments for Alzheimer's disease. Alzheimer's first robbed Uncle Bob of his short-term memory and then of his ability to care for himself. But I refused to let his disease cloud my memories of what an incredible person he was. These personal experiences instilled in me the empathy and motivation to dedicate my professional career to combating this most challenging disease.

memory loss, but depression, a loss of interest in pleasurable activities, a change in personality, increasing anxiety, a change in sleep patterns, or even a loss or decrease in the sense of smell. AD is a progressive disease with a wide range of severity. In fact, as you'll soon read, when AD first begins, there aren't any noticeable symptoms at all. As the disease advances, though, symptoms increase and become more significant, often including disorientation, difficulty communicating, behavioral shifts, and impaired judgment.

It's helpful to understand the symptoms in relation to the stages of AD in which they're usually seen. While over the years, scientists have proposed a number of ways to describe the progression of Alzheimer's disease, the model we use in our own practices is the one proposed by the National Institute on Aging and the Alzheimer's Association in 2011. This model reflects new findings in the research field, and more accurately portrays the disease as scientists currently understand it. It also takes into account modern innovations in clinical, imaging, and laboratory testing.

According to this new, more accurate model, there are three basic stages of AD:

- *Stage 1:* Preclinical Alzheimer's disease.

- *Stage 2:* Mild cognitive impairment (MCI) due to Alzheimer's disease.

- *Stage 3:* Dementia due to Alzheimer's disease.

We also use the term Stage 0, in which a person has no symptoms of memory loss, nor has that person begun to develop Alzheimer's disease in the brain. In Stage 0, it is unclear whether that person will develop AD in the future. In this stage—when people are most commonly in their twenties, thirties, forties, or fifties—we recommend making brain-healthy dietary and lifestyle choices that may help to *prevent* or *delay* the onset of the disease. In the following pages, we'll review the three basic stages of Alzheimer's disease itself, explaining how each stage is defined and detailing the symptoms that are most commonly associated with it.

Other Models for Diagnosing AD

Don't be surprised if your doctor uses terms other than the ones we've discussed to explain the various stages of Alzheimer's disease. Over the last three decades, doctors and scientists have developed a number of different models to help them understand and diagnose the stages of Alzheimer's disease. Some models had three stages; others, as many as seven. Until recently, the most commonly used model was the one presented in the *Diagnostic and Statistical Manual of Mental Disorders* (*DSM*). According to the *DSM,* in order to be diagnosed with AD, a person needed to show signs of new short-term memory problems, plus at least one of the following:

- *Aphasia:* Problems with language or speaking skills.

- *Apraxia:* Difficulty performing movements or tasks such as combing hair, brushing teeth, or driving.

- *Agnosia:* Difficulty recognizing common objects (remote control, pencil, coffee mug).

- *Loss of executive function:* Impaired judgment, problem solving, or thinking skills needed for everyday activities (such as planning a grocery shopping list).

STAGE 1   Preclinical Alzheimer's Disease

In the first stage of AD, a person shows no outward signs of the disease; memory and cognitive skills seem to be intact. Yet the person's brain has already begun to undergo certain changes that are associated with the development of Alzheimer's disease. These "hallmarks" of the disease are characteristic abnormalities that are typically observed in the brains of AD patients after death—abnormalities that are thought to contribute to the death or dysfunction of brain cells over time.

Over the years, scientists have focused on two particular hallmarks: beta-amyloid plaques and neurofibrillary or tau tangles. *Beta-amyloid plaques* are clumps of a protein called beta-amyloid that stick to the outsides of brain cells, possibly preventing them from commu-

For someone to be diagnosed with AD, these difficulties would also need to interfere with the normal activities of daily life, represent a decline from prior functioning, and occur with a gradual onset and slowly progressive course that could not be explained by any other condition (such as Parkinson's disease, thyroid dysfunction, the pseudodementia of depression, or substance-induced conditions).

Under this model, there were three different stages of AD. The disease was considered to advance from "mild" to "moderate" to "severe" AD. The main problem was that there was no clear consensus among physicians about when to use these terms. Some doctors used cognitive testing to determine the stage of AD, and others determined the severity of the disease based on the patient's ability to function on an everyday basis. In addition, this model didn't acknowledge the fact that the disease begins to develop before any symptoms even appear, and it didn't account for advances in testing (see page 41) that allow doctors to recognize the disease sooner.

Seeking to address these shortcomings, in 2011, doctors and scientists convened by the National Institute on Aging and the Alzheimer's Association developed the three-stage model described in this chapter. We use this model to diagnose AD because we feel it most accurately reflects our current understanding of the disease.

nicating with each other. Similarly, *tau tangles* involve strands of a protein called tau. Ordinarily, these protein strands help transport nutrients and other materials within your brain cells; in AD brains, they instead get snarled up, interfering with the cells' ability to function. Unable to function properly for various reasons, the brain cells eventually die.

But the accumulation of amyloid plaques and tau tangles aren't the only characteristic brain changes associated with the onset of Alzheimer's disease. Over the last few decades, scientists have discovered that many other changes take place. These changes are starting to receive more attention now. For example, scientists have noted that people with Alzheimer's disease have a reduced capacity to metabolize (use) glucose, a form of sugar that is the brain's primary source of fuel. This reduction in healthy glucose metabolism, known

Dr. Isaacson's Uncle Bob, Age Thirty-One

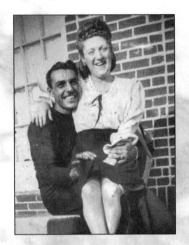

Uncle Bob entered the Navy during World War II and served in the South Pacific aboard the destroyer escort USS *Osmus*, where he was an anti-aircraft gunner and the ship's barber. After receiving an honorable discharge before the war's end, he opened a candy store in Brooklyn, New York. With things looking up, he and my Aunt Idy welcomed the arrival of their first child, my cousin Cynthia, in 1948.

Decades later, Uncle Bob's Navy training saved my life. When I was three years old, I fell into the pool at my Aunt Carol's house and disappeared under the water. Instinctively, Uncle Bob jumped in to rescue me. I appreciate all that he did to enable me to get where I am today!

as *glucose hypometabolism,* is significant because when brain cells are deprived of their main fuel source, they have a hard time functioning properly and eventually become damaged.

Scientists believe that these hallmark brain changes may begin twenty years or more before any symptoms of AD are visible. For - tunately, advances in laboratory testing and imaging have made it possible to detect these brain changes before memory loss begins. New tests look for *biomarkers,* which are measurable physiological, biochemical, and anatomic signs that suggest that these significant changes have occurred. Biomarkers help predict whether a person either has a disease or may develop it in the future. For example, certain biomarkers point to the existence of amyloid plaques. Additional biomarkers announce other changes in the brain, bloodstream, eyes, skin, and fluid surrounding the brain that have been associated with the development of AD. If tests indicate that these biomarkers are present, it is likely that you have a greater risk of developing Alzheimer's disease.

What Is "Normal" Brain Aging?

As we age, our brains ordinarily undergo certain physical and chemical changes. The severity of these changes may depend on a variety of genetic and environmental risk factors over our lifespans. Brain cells age at different rates, parts of the brain shrink, and the chemicals that help the neurons communicate increase or decline. Not surprisingly, as our brains change, our cognitive abilities change, too.

The problem is, scientists disagree about which of these brain changes can truly be considered "normal"—that is, expected as part of the aging process—and which changes occur as the result of other chronic conditions and disorders, such as Alzheimer's disease. This is because studies increasingly point to anomalies: patients with brain changes associated with AD who show no signs of cognitive decline, and patients with no brain changes associated with AD who do have cognitive decline.

Consider one of the so-called hallmarks of Alzheimer's disease, beta-amyloid plaques. In an ongoing study at the University of California at Irvine, Dr. Claudia Kawas and her colleagues have been investigating the factors that allow people to live to age ninety and beyond. On average, one-third of the individuals in this study had dementia, one-third had some form of cognitive impairment without dementia, and one-third were normal. When researchers looked at the brains of the study participants, they found that nearly 50 percent had amyloid plaques. Clearly, certain people were able to avoid AD and maintain higher levels of cognitive functioning despite the presence of a substance many believe to be a sign of AD. This suggests that beta-amyloid may not necessarily be as significant to the diagnosis of AD as previously thought—or that other factors might play roles in both accelerating decline or protecting the brain against AD.

In short, scientists have a long way to go before they are reliably able to distinguish between "normal" brain aging and brain changes that result from more deep-seated conditions. We still don't quite know why some people experience what's known as "successful" cognitive aging—aging with no changes in memory or thinking skills—and others go on to develop Alzheimer's disease. Research is ongoing, as this kind of knowledge will be invaluable, potentially allowing doctors to diagnose, prevent, and treat AD earlier and more accurately.

Similarly, in place of more invasive and often expensive lab or radiology tests, more and more doctors are using very specific types of memory tests to look for "cognitive biomarkers." A lower-than-expected score on a memory test can be considered an early sign of AD. Some doctors think that these tests are currently better and more accurate in detecting AD than the blood-based biomarker tests. Increasingly, these detailed memory tests are administered by neurologists using highly sensitive computer programs. If you'd like to try some examples of these kinds of tests, go to www.AlzU.org and sign up for a free account; samples are available on the Activities tab. (Also see the discussion of diagnostic tests on page 40.)

Biomarker testing has changed the ways in which medical professionals look at Alzheimer's disease. As testing techniques for bio-

Is It Alzheimer's Prevention or Alzheimer's Treatment?

The future of Alzheimer's research lies in being able to identify patients in the first preclinical stage of the disease. Doctors agree that this stage is the ideal time to suggest that people make brain-healthy choices that can reduce the risk of Alzheimer's disease and even delay its onset. But they differ as to whether these medical interventions should be considered treatment or prevention. Because patients in this first stage of the disease do not appear to have symptoms of cognitive impairment, many doctors consider the lifestyle modifications that they recommend to be preventive of the disease. But this is not entirely accurate. After all, biomarker tests can make it clear that the disease is already present, regardless of whether there are symptoms. As a result, we think it's more accurate to consider any interventions undertaken in this stage as *treatment.* That is to say, by the time a biomarker test indicates the presence of the disease, it's too late to actually prevent the disease from occurring altogether, but it's certainly not too late to slow the disease and keep it from progressing to Stages 2 or 3. We reserve the term *prevention* for people in Stage 0 who have not developed preclinical AD—people with no symptoms of memory loss and no biomarker evidence of AD. These people would generally be classified as normal.

Dr. Isaacson's Uncle Bob, Age Forty-Five

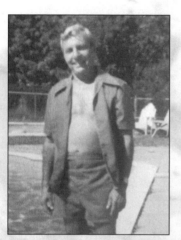

While running his candy store, my Uncle Bob often helped our Uncle Morris with house painting, learning another trade that he enjoyed. When he realized he could make more money and work fewer hours painting than he could selling candy, he started his own painting, wallpapering, and general contracting business. He was a "gentleman painter," leaving home every morning wearing pressed slacks and a collared shirt. He would change into his painter's overalls at the job but return home in his nice clothes, as handsome as when he had left that morning. Oh yes, he was a proud and dignified man.

During the period that Uncle Bob was developing his business, my cousins Frank and Guy were born. The family moved into a larger apartment in Brooklyn. Things were going well. But what nobody realized was that by time Bob was forty-five, the very first processes related to Alzheimer's disease had begun in his brain. On the outside, he seemed healthy, active, and successful, with normal memory and thinking skills. Yet on the inside, preclinical AD (Stage 1) was just starting to take hold.

markers become more accurate and sophisticated, doctors will be able to identify the disease in patients much earlier than they have been able to do in the past. This is incredibly significant, because the sooner the disease is identified, the sooner the patient will know to take steps to improve brain health, if he or she is not already doing so!

STAGE 2 Mild Cognitive Impairment Due to Alzheimer's

The second stage of Alzheimer's disease is called mild cognitive impairment (MCI) due to Alzheimer's disease. *Mild cognitive impairment* is commonly characterized by changes in thinking skills that have not yet impacted the patient's daily life. Individuals may have recognizable problems with memory, language, thinking skills, or judgment, but these problems do not limit their ability to carry out everyday activities. This means that people with MCI are still able to work, drive, prepare meals, and shop, much as they have done before. In general, mild cognitive impairment does not necessarily have to be caused by Alzheimer's disease; it can be prompted by a variety of different underlying conditions, including depression, thyroid dysfunction, vitamin B_{12} deficiency, or head trauma. It can be challenging for doctors to identify the source of a person's MCI, but more detailed cognitive testing can help. Most commonly, doctors find that a person has MCI due to AD when problems with short-term memory appear in combination with other cognitive deficits that can be identified during testing, such as difficulties with language or executive function (decision-making).

Once a patient has been formally diagnosed with MCI, the chances that he or she will progress from MCI to a more advanced stage of memory loss called *dementia* increase by 10 to 15 percent each year. While there are many potential causes for dementia, by far the most common is Alzheimer's disease. Still, it's important to note that while many individuals with MCI eventually develop dementia due to Alzheimer's disease, more than half do not. Some go on to develop other types of dementia, and others—those for whom the cause of MCI is unclear—may even regain normal memory.

Because this is the stage of AD in which symptoms are first seen, it is often during this stage that doctors are able to diagnose AD. Common symptoms of MCI include:

- Memory problems that can be recognized by the individual, family members, and/or medical professionals.

- Not knowing the right sequence of steps to finish a task.

- Inability to access previously high-functioning decision-making abilities.

- Difficulty retaining material recently read.

- Occasionally losing objects.

- Increasing difficulty with organizational skills.

At this point in the disease progression, biomarker changes are similar to those found in preclinical AD, though they become more pronounced and even easier to detect. Patients accumulate more amyloid plaques, and glucose hypometabolism also increases. These biomarker changes may be tracked over time using a variety of methods, including radiology (a PET scan, for example). Testing is still uncommon, however, and not done routinely for disease management in the typical patient. At this time, biomarker changes are usually tracked only in research trials.

Dr. Isaacson's Uncle Bob, Age Sixty-Six

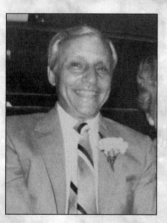

With his family and business flourishing, and many commercial contracts coming in, my Uncle Bob and Aunt Idy bought a brand-new two-family home in the newly developed area of Brooklyn called Canarsie. Trying to get more serious about his health, Uncle Bob stopped smoking cigarettes. But at age fifty-three, Uncle Bob had a massive heart attack while working at a neighbor's house. Somehow he made his way home, clutching his chest, sweating, and vomiting. His son Frank ran for the doctor down the block. Uncle Bob nearly died in the ambulance ride to the hospital, but was brought back by paramedics. We bless that doctor and those paramedics to this day.

From that moment on, Uncle Bob's world was different. He changed his diet, stayed on his medications, kept busy with small projects, and continued walking Brutus, his Saint Bernard. By the age of sixty-six, Bob was spending summer weekends in the country with his family. For the most part, life was good. Yet several people close to Bob had begun to notice that he was having a few "senior moments," misplacing objects, forgetting an appointment, or repeating a question here and there. Attributing this to just another part of normal aging, Bob did not seek medical attention. But Uncle Bob had now entered Stage 2 Alzheimer's disease, or MCI due to Alzheimer's disease.

The Difference Between Age-Related Cognitive Decline and Mild Cognitive Impairment Due to AD

As we explained on page 13, our brains undergo certain physical and chemical changes as part of the natural aging process. As our brains change, our cognitive abilities change, too. This is why, for example, a child can learn a new language much more easily than a college student or older adult. Research shows that older adults process information less efficiently than healthy young adults, due in part to the fact that more brain cells in older people have sustained more damage over more time.

But just because your ability to learn may be reduced doesn't mean that you necessarily have dementia. Typically, we refer to the set of minor cognitive changes that occur as a natural part of the aging process as *age-associated cognitive decline.* The symptoms of age-associated cognitive decline may include intermittent memory loss, word-finding difficulties, and a slower speed of thinking. When the cognitive changes are isolated to difficulties with memory, this condition is sometimes referred to as *age-related memory loss.*

How do we know that a slight lapse or senior moment is associated with this "normal" age-associated cognitive decline, then, and that it's not a sign of mild cognitive impairment or Alzheimer's disease? Misplacing objects and forgetting appointments are common symptoms of early AD—but they also happen to people who don't have AD. And a lot of the time, what we think of as forgetfulness is actually the result of not paying attention in the first place. For those of us who lead busy lives with constant distractions (phones ringing, text messages coming in, children shouting in the background), it's easy to lose track of things or to fail to take in what our friends, spouses, or parents are telling us. But when a person continually misplaces objects or loses them altogether, or when that person constantly tells stories or asks questions over and over again with no recollection or realization of this repetition, it may be a sign of something more serious, like early AD.

Clearly, it can be difficult to distinguish between "normal" age-associated cognitive impairment (or just inattention) and Alzheimer's disease. This problem is compounded by the fact that doctors don't always agree on what "normal" brain aging and cognitive change *is*. As a result, many cases of AD go unrecognized early on, as the symptoms are considered to be benign signs of aging. Still, there are some ways to know whether memory loss is significant. For example, if you're over the age of thirty, it's normal to forget the name of an acquaintance you haven't seen in a long time. The name will be on the tip of your tongue, and later, it will come back to you in a snap. For people who have AD, that moment often doesn't arrive. It's important to realize that sleep deprivation, stressful life events, side effects from a medication, or a severe medical illness can mimic the signs of AD.

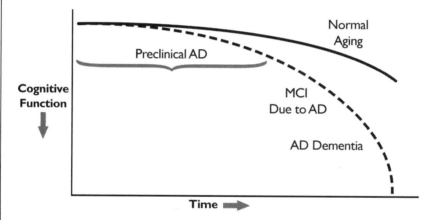

Figure 1.1. The Progression of Cognitive Decline in AD and in Normal Aging

Figure 1.1 illustrates the difference between normal age-associated cognitive decline and cognitive decline due to AD. The solid line shows how cognitive function declines gradually over time in normal aging, and the dotted line shows how cognitive function declines over the three stages of AD—first slowly, and then more rapidly. It's important to note that cognitive decline may not be apparent in the preclinical years of AD, although detailed cognitive testing can reveal some changes. As the graphic shows, cognitive decline tends to be more detectable between Stages 1 and 2 of AD.

STAGE 3   Dementia Due to Alzheimer's Disease

Stage 3 is called *dementia due to AD,* and it is characterized by memory loss and other cognitive impairments that interfere with the activities of daily living. An individual with Alzheimer's dementia may need assistance in completing everyday tasks such as cooking, bathing, and dressing. Because the symptoms of Alzheimer's dementia worsen over time, doctors now divide this stage of AD into three distinct phases: mild, moderate, and severe dementia.

Mild Dementia Due to Alzheimer's Disease

Many people are first diagnosed with AD after they've already reached this earliest phase of dementia. The signs of cognitive impairment become clear and unmistakable to friends, family, and medical professionals.

Common symptoms of mild Alzheimer's dementia include:

- Forgetting recent events (memory loss severe enough to interfere with daily living).

- Repeating the same story over and over again.

- Increasing difficulty performing complex tasks such as balancing a checkbook, planning a big dinner party, or managing household finances.

- Mild depression.

- Moodiness or withdrawn behavior that usually worsens in challenging situations such as large social gatherings.

- Difficulty in formulating and expressing thoughts.

Moderate Dementia Due to Alzheimer's Disease

As cognition declines further, people in this stage of dementia may begin to need assistance with daily activities and self-care.

Common symptoms of moderate Alzheimer's dementia include:

- Worsening and increasingly noticeable gaps in both memory and thinking.

- Difficulty in remembering simple information such as an address or telephone number.

- Disorientation and confusion regarding the date or current surroundings; may get lost.

- Difficulty dressing properly (selecting seasonally appropriate clothing, putting on clothing).

- More significant changes in personality and behavior.

- Some difficulty recalling personal history.

- Inability to recall names.

- Sleep pattern disturbances: restlessness or insomnia at night, sleeping too much during the day.

- Increasingly more disoriented; individuals may wander.

- Help needed with daily activities like using the toilet.

Severe Dementia Due to Alzheimer's Disease

In the last phase of dementia due to AD, cognition has declined so significantly that an individual is increasingly unable to function independently and may have additional physical problems and restrictions.

Common symptoms of severe Alzheimer's dementia include:

- Help required for most personal daily needs.

- Difficulty communicating.

- Swallowing may become impaired.

- More significant personality and behavior changes; may become suspicious or aggressive, or have repetitive compulsive behavior.

As we'll explain in the section on diagnosis, there is no standardized approach to determining the exact stage or phase of AD to which an individual may belong. Physicians lack consensus about when to use the terms mild, moderate, or severe dementia due to AD. Some physicians use the results of cognitive testing, and others determine the severity based on how the patient is functioning on an everyday basis. Most important is that the disease be diagnosed as soon as possible. We are strong advocates for early diagnosis, and we advise peo-

Dr. Isaacson's Uncle Bob, Age Seventy-Two

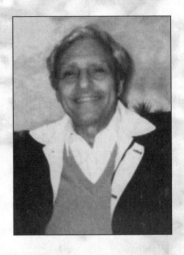

In 1986, with all their children out of the house, Uncle Bob and Aunt Idy decided to sell their home in Canarsie and retire to south Florida. Shortly after the move, Aunt Idy was diagnosed with breast cancer, devastating Uncle Bob and our entire family. After a rough road, they welcomed their first granddaughter, Ciara. Her birth gave Aunt Idy a newfound strength. Still, as Idy's health declined, so did Bob's mental state. After Aunt Idy passed, Uncle Bob began to show more and more signs of stress-related dementia, as it was called at the time.

Uncle Bob lived alone in their condo for a few years, but as his mental state started to slip and his memory faltered, the decision to consider an assisted living facility was made. Uncle Bob really appreciated the social environment of his new home, and did very well there; in fact, he often took care of other residents in need. He enjoyed the entertainment, sing-alongs, and frequent visits from his daughter Cynthia, who lived close by and often took him out shopping, to the beach, and to dinner. Despite his memory decline, he never forgot any of the words of his favorite songs, especially those by Frank Sinatra.

Eventually, Uncle Bob was diagnosed with Alzheimer's disease, which we now refer to as Stage 3 AD, and which also claimed the lives of every one of his four siblings. Uncle Bob loved life and lived it to the fullest, enjoying every moment as though it was his last. He was the patriarch who gave his children the strength to live on. He passed at home on April 21, 2002.

ple to seek medical attention when symptoms first begin—and to make brain-healthy choices even before that point. As we've said before, the earlier a doctor can diagnose AD, the earlier the disease can be treated. And the earlier the disease is treated, the better the patient will do.

THE CAUSES OF AD

Scientists do not yet know what causes AD. Alzheimer's disease is very complex, and research indicates that it is probably set in motion by a variety of factors, including genetics, lifestyle, and environment. In about 5 percent of all AD cases, the disease is directly caused by mutations in one of three genes: amyloid precursor protein (APP), presenilin-1 (PS-1), and presenilin-2 (PS-2). People who have inherited these "deterministic" genetic variations are virtually guaranteed to develop AD, and will usually be diagnosed earlier in life—before the age of sixty-five, and sometimes as young as thirty or forty. For this reason, this rare form of AD is called *familial* or *early-onset Alzheimer's.*

For the most part, it's still not clear what causes the vast majority of late-onset AD cases. In an effort to understand why Alzheimer's develops, some scientists have considered the possibility that it is caused by the two hallmarks of the disease mentioned earlier, beta-amyloid plaques and tau tangles. As we have explained, in Alzheimer's patients, these two protein formations typically occur in excess, building up and possibly causing damage in the areas of the brain that are responsible for memory.

Clearly, these hallmarks are heavily associated with the progression of AD. But research increasingly indicates that plaques and tangles play a more indirect role in the disease, or may even be a result of another disease process that precedes their formation. In fact, some scientists feel that the development of AD may occur independently of amyloid deposition. They suggest that the progression of AD might actually be related to glucose hypometabolism. In turn, this glucose hypometabolism may be caused by *mitochondrial dysfunction,* a problem in which the mitochondria (or "batteries" of the brain cells) have difficulty processing energy. For reasons that are not yet clear, mitochondrial dysfunction not only causes glucose hypometabolism, but may additionally contribute to a condition called oxidative stress. In oxidative stress, cells that are deprived of sufficient energy find it difficult to detoxify, potentially leading to cell damage and injury. As you'll see in this book, some of the most powerful therapies that may improve mitochondrial function and reduce oxidative stress also happen to be among the simplest to implement. By making easy changes to your diet and lifestyle, you may be able to protect your brain.

Significantly, research has shown that beta-amyloid proteins can also be found in the brains of people showing no symptoms of AD— both younger people and normal adults over the age of sixty-five. While it is not known whether these people will yet go on to develop Alzheimer's, the fact that beta-amyloid can be found in both normal and AD brains suggests that this protein might not instigate the disease, but might instead be a byproduct or symptom of a deeper-rooted cause.

Although scientists are currently unable to pinpoint exact causes of AD, they have been able to identify several risk factors that increase the chance that a person will develop the disease.

RISK FACTORS

Risk factors are traits, characteristics, behaviors, exposures, or conditions that increase the likelihood that a person will develop a certain disease. There are two types of risk factors: modifiable and nonmodifiable. *Modifiable risk factors* are risk factors you can change or eliminate. For example, smoking is a modifiable risk factor for lung cancer; you can decide to quit, and if you do quit, your risk of developing lung cancer will decrease dramatically. By contrast, *nonmodifiable risk factors* are beyond your control, like genetics or family history. If both of your parents developed heart disease at an early age, you are more likely to also develop heart disease early, because while you may be able to take steps to decrease your overall risk, there's nothing you can do to reduce the family risk factor.

Fortunately, great progress has been made over the last decade in determining the many modifiable and nonmodifiable risk factors involved in the development of Alzheimer's disease. An extensive review of all of the risk factors for AD is beyond the scope of this book, but in this section, we'll outline the major risk factors that deserve consideration. If you want to learn more, we encourage you to check out the AlzRisk AD Epidemiology Database, a frequently updated website that provides comprehensive coverage of the latest information on all Alzheimer's risk factors. (Turn to page 230 of the Resources list.)

We'd like to make it clear that although a risk factor may increase the likelihood that a person will develop AD, it does not mean that the individual will definitely develop the disease. The goal of this book is to demonstrate that there are many steps you can take to reduce your risk of developing Alzheimer's disease and to enjoy healthy memory and cognition for years to come. And the first step in reducing your risk is knowing what your risk factors are.

Age

Age is the number-one risk factor for Alzheimer's disease. Generally speaking, the older you are, the more likely you are to develop Alzheimer's disease. According to the Alzheimer's Association, the risk of developing Alzheimer's disease doubles nearly every five years after the age of sixty-five. By age eighty-five, the risk of developing Alzheimer's is well over 35 percent. Why does age matter? As we explained earlier, your brain cells naturally sustain damage over time as part of the aging process. As you live longer, your brain cells sustain more damage, and a greater number of brain cells cease to function normally. Aging is also associated with an increased risk of circulatory problems. We depend on the cardiovascular system to bring oxygen and nutrients to our brain cells; when this system is weakened, damaged, or impaired, our brain cells don't get these essential substances and can die.

That being said, just because you're getting older doesn't mean you'll develop AD. Many people live beyond the age of ninety with relatively little or no cognitive decline. By taking steps to preserve and protect your memory, you will greatly increase the chances that you will remain cognitively healthy throughout your life.

25

Family History

One of the most common questions we get about AD is, "If I have a family history of Alzheimer's disease, am I more likely to develop it myself?" Before we answer, we usually remind people that AD is a very common condition regardless of family history; everybody's risk increases with advancing age. That being said, family history is considered a risk factor for AD, because there are specific genes that can be passed from parents to children that raise the likelihood of developing Alzheimer's. If you have one or more first-degree family

---

Assessing AD Risk at the Alzheimer's Prevention Clinic

In 2013, Dr. Isaacson founded the Alzheimer's Prevention Clinic (APC) at Weill Cornell Medicine and NewYork-Presbyterian—the first health center in the United States devoted to AD prevention in a clinical setting. The primary goals of the clinic are to employ preventative measures to address AD in patients before symptoms become apparent and to suggest evidence-based therapies meant to delay the progression toward dementia in those who have already been diagnosed with MCI or AD. Patients range in age from twenty-seven to ninety-one—you can never be too young or too old to think about AD prevention. Most of our patients are people who are considered "cognitively healthy"—that is, they have no symptoms of memory loss—although they often have at least one family member who has been diagnosed with AD. We also see patients who have age-related cognitive decline, Stage 1 or 2 AD, or cognitive issues caused by other health conditions. Using the latest research and the most current diagnostic tools available, Dr. Isaacson and his colleagues formulate a personalized plan of action for each patient to effectively reduce the likelihood that he or she will develop symptoms of Alzheimer's disease.

To do this, we first employ a variety of methods to assess AD risk. Using a very detailed questionnaire, we take a comprehensive medical and personal history. For example, we ask each patient about past medical problems; years of higher education; and dietary, exercise, and

members—a parent or sibling, for example—who developed AD, you may be more likely to develop it, too, perhaps more so if the affected relative developed the disease at an early age (usually before age sixty).

Genetics

Clearly, genetics are a significant risk factor for AD. As you learned earlier (see page 23), a very small group of people who carry at least one of three genetic mutations are virtually guaranteed to develop

sleep patterns. We also ask how many family members have been diagnosed with AD, and the age at which each person was diagnosed. After completing the initial questionnaire, patients complete an online course about AD prevention that our team created on Alzheimer's Universe (www.AlzU.org), which is also free for the public to join.

Then, we do a physical workup. We measure vital signs and a number of other basic factors, including body fat percentage and waist circumference. Based on all this initial information, we are able to use previously established algorithms (step-by-step procedures) to determine a variety of AD risk scores. We then use laboratory studies (including blood work) to look closely at a number of inflammatory, metabolic, nutritional, and other biomarkers associated with AD, such as levels of cholesterol, blood sugar, insulin, vitamins, and omega-3 fatty acids. We also run a battery of tests to evaluate cognitive functioning. In addition, patients in the clinic have the option of genetic testing. It's important to note that while doctors generally do not use genetic testing to assess the risk of AD, in this highly specialized clinic, we use these tests to help create personalized treatment and prevention strategies for our patients.

After taking all of these different factors into account, the treating neurologist puts together a comprehensive therapy program that addresses the individual's risk. As the patient continues on this program, the series of tests is repeated on a routine basis to evaluate how the recommendations are working. The patient also uses our AD-Nutrition Tracking System to help assess progress.

early-onset Alzheimer's disease. But researchers have also identified a gene that may be associated with a higher risk for late-onset AD. This gene is called *apolipoprotein epsilon,* or APOE, and scientists believe its main job is to help regulate cholesterol transport and metabolism.

There are three different forms of the APOE gene: APOE2, APOE3, and APOE4. Briefly, you get one copy of the APOE gene from your mother and another copy from your father. Most people, or up to 60 percent of all Americans, receive the APOE3 form from both parents. Comparatively fewer people receive the APOE2 and APOE4 forms. Between 20 and 30 percent of all Americans will inherit one or more copies of APOE4; studies show that these people may have a greater risk of developing AD. Studies indicate that between 40 and 65 percent of all Alzheimer's patients have at least one copy of the APOE4 gene. Conversely, the 10 to 20 percent of Americans who inherit one or more copies of APOE2 may have a reduced risk of developing AD.

It's very important to note that the presence of these genes does not definitively predict whether you will (or will not) develop AD. Many people who carry the APOE4 gene never develop Alzheimer's disease, and many without the APOE4 gene do develop AD. For this reason, most physicians discourage their patients from undergoing genetic testing for APOE. The significance of the results is still too unclear for this kind of data to be reliably useful in general medical practice.

Moreover, there are a number of ways in which you can modify your lifestyle to win the tug-of-war with your genes, mitigating their negative impact on your risk of developing Alzheimer's disease. For example, research shows that people with the APOE4 gene who engage in regular exercise can reduce amyloid deposits in the brain so that their levels are equivalent to the levels in people who *don't* have the APOE4 gene. (See page 178 to learn more about exercise and AD.)

Gender

Women appear to be more likely than men to develop Alzheimer's disease; they account for about two-thirds of all AD patients in the United States. This figure may be partially explained by the fact that women generally tend to live longer—and, as you learned earlier, the longer you live, the more likely you are to develop AD. That being said, gender may, in fact, have a bearing on AD risk. Recent studies suggest that women who carry the APOE4 gene are more likely than men with the gene to develop Alzheimer's disease. Whether sex affects AD risk in those who do not carry the gene is still in debate. Additionally, some scientists believe that different hormone levels between the sexes may also play a role in determining AD risk. Clearly, more research is needed.

Race and Ethnicity

Some research indicates that African Americans and Latinos are more likely than whites of the same age to develop AD, and that they are also more likely to develop AD earlier in life. By one estimate, African Americans are twice as likely and Latinos one and a half times as likely as whites to develop AD. However, this disparity may be explained by differences in rates of health conditions such as high blood pressure, heart disease, and diabetes. African Americans and Latinos have higher rates of these disorders, which, as you'll see, act as independent risk factors for AD.

While there may or may not be a genetic basis for differences in AD incidence rates between racial groups, it is important that people of all backgrounds be attentive to the risks and symptoms of Alzheimer's. No matter what your cultural heritage, you can and should take steps to minimize your risks and make your lifestyle more brain-healthy.

Cardiovascular Disease and Related Problems

Cardiovascular (heart) disease is the number-one cause of death in the United States, making it a devastating condition in its own right. But scientists now believe that cardiovascular disease may also have vast implications for the development of Alzheimer's disease. Simply put, the health of your brain is linked to the health of your heart! The brain needs oxygen and nutrients in order to function normally, and it gets these essential materials from blood, which is pumped through blood vessels by the heart. If the heart and blood vessels aren't healthy—for example, if the heart is weak or the blood vessels are blocked—blood won't flow steadily or quickly enough to meet the oxygen and nutrient demands of the brain. Deprived of these vital substances, brain cells begin to die, cognitive abilities can be compromised, and dementia can develop over time.

Because of the close association between heart health and brain health, many factors that increase the risk of cardiovascular disease also increase the risk of Alzheimer's and other dementias. As we mentioned earlier, Latinos and African Americans—two populations that have higher rates of cardiovascular disease—are particularly vulnerable to AD. Fortunately, most of these risk factors are modifiable. If you have any of the cardiovascular risk factors that are discussed beginning on page 31, you may want to consult with your doctor to create a treatment plan that can get your heart health back on track. Doctors who specialize in preventative cardiology are usually open to taking a more comprehensive approach to reducing the risk of heart attacks and other major health events.

The relationship between cardiovascular and cognitive health has been well established. In the Northern Manhattan Study, Dr. Ralph Sacco and his team at the Neurological Institute have been investigating stroke risk factors in different racial and ethnic groups in New York for more than twenty years. As part of their research, Dr. Sacco's team has also explored the association between stroke risk factors and cognitive decline.

Based on their research, Dr. Sacco and his colleagues created a model, the Global Vascular Risk Score (GVRS). The GVRS considers the factors that contribute to vascular (blood vessel) damage in the brain—such as obesity, high blood pressure, and alcohol consumption—and is primarily seen as a way of evaluating how likely a person is to have a stroke. But because vascular damage is itself a major risk factor for brain shrinkage and cognitive decline, the GVRS can be a useful tool in helping doctors determine and modify cardiovascular risk that may also adversely affect the brain. To discover your GVRS, you can use the online GVRS calculator at http://neurology.med .miami.edu/gvr. As always, you should talk to your doctor about your results. Keep in mind, however, that your score doesn't have an exact bearing on whether or not you will develop cognitive decline or AD. The Northern Manhattan Study found that a fifth of all participants who had vascular damage never had any symptoms of cognitive impairment significant enough to warrant medical attention. Although cardiovascular disease and its related conditions obviously play significant roles in determining each person's risk for AD, they are far from the only factors at work.

The following discussions provide more information on cardiovascular risk factors that also increase the chance of developing AD. These modifiable risk factors can be managed in a variety of ways, including lifestyle changes; medications; and, especially, dietary modifications.

High Cholesterol

Cholesterol itself isn't necessarily a bad thing. Cholesterol performs a number of important roles in the brain; among other things, it helps maintain the structure and functioning of your brain cells.

High cholesterol levels, however—particularly high levels of low-density lipoprotein (LDL), or "bad" cholesterol—are linked to a higher risk of both heart disease and Alzheimer's disease. Studies have shown that people who have high LDL cholesterol levels are more likely to have greater brain deposits of beta-amyloid protein, one of the hallmarks of AD. It's not clear, though, whether the high cholesterol levels *cause* the greater formation of beta-amyloid plaques, or potentially whether the high levels represent the body's attempts to *protect* the brain against AD.

In addition, high LDL cholesterol levels are linked to atherosclerosis, a narrowing or hardening of the arteries. Atherosclerosis impairs blood circulation, and as a result can also impair the proper functioning of the brain, which depends on blood vessels to transport oxygen and nutrients.

Further study is warranted to explain the relationship between cholesterol levels and AD. New research also suggests that genetics may influence the way people react to cholesterol, adding new complexity to the issue. In the meantime, we recommend that people with high levels of LDL cholesterol and low levels of HDL cholesterol—high-density lipoprotein, or "good" cholesterol—see a doctor to begin a treatment program. In his practice, Dr. Isaacson closely follows both LDL and HDL cholesterol levels in his patients. He also measures the particle size of these cholesterol molecules. Very small and dense LDL particles (as opposed to large and fluffy particles) raise the risk of cardiovascular disease by increasing inflammation and contributing to blood clot formation. While there is some disagreement about the use of statin drugs, your doctor may recommend these or other cholesterol-reducing medications—as well as supplements such as niacin and omega-3 fatty acids, and lifestyle changes such as diet and exercise—to help you reach healthier blood levels.

Obesity in Midlife

The bulk of current research suggests that obesity—usually defined as body mass index (BMI) greater than 30 (see the inset on page 52)—may increase the risk of Alzheimer's disease and other forms of dementia or cognitive decline later in life, particularly when people are overweight in their forties and fifties. The association may be indirect, as people who are obese tend to have higher rates of LDL cholesterol, diabetes, physical inactivity, and cardiovascular disease—all health problems that independently raise the risk of AD. But new studies indicate that obesity may directly contribute to Alzheimer's disease, as well. For one thing, people who carry certain variants of the fat mass and obesity-associated (FTO) gene are more likely to develop Alzheimer's, especially when they also carry the APOE4 gene. In addition, the FTO gene seems to be linked to reduced brain volume. That is, people who have the FTO gene tend to have certain regions of their brain atrophy, or shrink, much more significantly than do people without the gene. With less brain matter available, cognitive function is impaired.

On the other hand, one recent large-scale study suggests that people who are obese are *less* likely to develop dementia. And some studies show that older adults who are *underweight* (having a BMI lower than 18.5) are more likely to develop AD than both people who are of normal weight and those who are a little overweight. There is also evidence that weight loss in older adults can be considered a symptom of Alzheimer's disease, which is possibly linked to one of the metabolic disturbances associated with the disorder.

There is still much work to be done to unravel the connection between body weight and AD. That being said, most of the relevant research indicates the importance of maintaining a healthy, normal weight. As you'll see in the next chapter and beyond, the key to a healthy weight—and a healthy mind—is diet.

Diabetes

Diabetes—particularly type 2 diabetes—is associated with a higher risk of Alzheimer's disease. By some estimates, diabetics are as much as twice as likely as nondiabetics to develop AD. Scientists are still working to understand the precise link between the two diseases, but some hypotheses have been formed. A primary theory has to do with the fact that diabetes is characterized by *insulin resistance,* a condition in which the body manufactures a hormone called insulin but is unable to respond to it properly. Insulin's main jobs are to help your cells take in glucose, the simple sugar that is the body's primary energy source, and to clear excess glucose out of the bloodstream after the body has absorbed all the energy it needs. Persistently elevated glucose levels can directly cause a number of problems, including cardiovascular disease, nerve conditions, and a decreased ability to fight infection. At the same time, the body produces more and more insulin to clear the high levels of glucose, potentially leading to detrimental inflammatory effects on the brain.

Insulin is essential to a number of brain processes, playing a role in memory formation and regulating a neurotransmitter called acetylcholine, a special chemical that allows brain cells to communicate with one another. Insulin also helps maintain the blood vessels that feed the brain, supporting the circulation of oxygen and nutrients. With insulin resistance, these functions are undermined, potentially leading to cognitive decline and memory loss. Interestingly, different areas of the brain may become more insulin resistant than others—research suggests that the hippocampus, the brain's memory center, may be particularly prone to insulin resistance. In addition, some studies indicate that insulin resistance is associated with a higher growth rate of beta-amyloid plaques, one of the hallmarks of AD.

While more research still needs to be done to explain the exact connection between diabetes, insulin resistance, and AD, the evidence supporting those associations is strong. Fortunately, many cases of diabetes—and, to some extent, Alzheimer's—can be managed, delayed, or possibly prevented with careful attention to diet and lifestyle. If you already have diabetes, are prediabetic, or are at risk of developing diabetes, talk to your doctor. Your body and mind will thank you.

Blood Pressure Problems

There is conflicting evidence about the role of high and low blood pressure in the development of Alzheimer's disease. High blood pressure in midlife (one's forties and fifties) is associated with a higher risk of Alzheimer's disease and other forms of dementia. Like high cholesterol and diabetes, high blood pressure increases the risk of AD by damaging blood vessels and thus impairing the flow of blood to the brain. Without enough of the oxygen and nutrients ordinarily brought by the blood, brain cells die, setting the stage for cognitive decline and Alzheimer's.

That being said, *low* blood pressure later in life (age seventy and older) may also increase the chances of cognitive decline or AD. In 2003, researchers at the University of California at Irvine began a long-term study to discover what factors allow people to live to age ninety and beyond. According to results of this ongoing "90+ Study," one of the factors that contribute to successful aging—aging without cognitive impairment or dementia—is actually *higher* blood pressure. There are two possible explanations for why this might reduce the risk of dementia. One is that low blood pressure makes it more difficult for the brain to receive an adequate flow of oxygen and nutrients, and thus contributes to brain deterioration over time. The other possibility is that it isn't the high blood pressure that protects against AD; rather, it is the medications used to treat this condition (calcium channel blockers, angiotensin receptor blockers, and ACE-inhibitors) that may deliver benefits to the brain.

By maintaining well-controlled, healthy blood pressure, you may be able to delay brain aging and preserve memory function for the future. We recommend keeping track of your blood pressure readings over time—for your convenience, we've provided some helpful tools online at www.AlzheimersDiet.com/alzu. Most doctors recommend a variety of lifestyle changes to control blood pressure. In addition to following the dietary guidelines provided in this book, if you have hypertension, you may want to talk to your doctor about reducing your salt intake or taking a prescription blood pressure medication.

Inadequate Physical Activity

Some studies show that people who are not physically active have a higher risk for AD and other forms of dementia. Generally, scientists agree that physical activity is one of the most protective factors for AD, indirectly reducing the risk of dementia by helping to maintain the health of the cardiovascular system, and thereby ensuring that there is good blood circulation of nutrients and oxygen to the brain. Importantly, physical activity has also been shown to *directly reduce amyloid levels in the brain,* and may also stimulate the growth of brain cells and the development of new connections between those brain cells. For these reasons, a lack of physical activity can be detrimental to the health of the brain.

There is a simple way to eliminate this particular risk factor for AD: Get more exercise! To keep your brain in good condition, it is essential that you stay or become physically active. For more information on using exercise to help prevent AD, see page 178.

Smoking

Not surprisingly, smoking is considered a risk factor for Alzheimer's disease, just as it is for many other serious disorders. Smoking damages the heart and blood vessels, making it harder for blood to reach the brain.

If you smoke, try to quit—there are many organizations and support groups that will help you kick the habit. And if you don't smoke now, don't start!

Head Injuries

Evidence suggests that head injuries involving loss of consciousness (such as a concussion) can increase the risk of AD, especially when the trauma is severe, suffered later in life, or occurs in people who carry the APOE4 gene. Scientists believe that serious brain injuries directly damage or kill brain cells, leading to cognitive impairment.

These injuries may also cause inflammation and encourage the development of brain pathology, such as tau tangles.

To reduce the impact of head injuries, it is always advisable to wear a protective helmet when engaging in certain activities, such as riding a bike. As research increasingly indicates that full-contact sports such as football, hockey, and wrestling may have serious consequences for the brains of the participating athletes, some colleges have begun to implement stricter rules for sports practices and events in an effort to reduce the possibility of head trauma. For example, certain schools limit the number or duration of full-contact practices; others have started limiting full-contact football practices; and rules are constantly being implemented to ensure that when athletes sustain any form of head trauma, they are immediately evaluated and advised to avoid further activity until they have been cleared by a qualified medical professional.

Heavy Metal Exposure

Some scientists have explored the possibility that heavy metals might also cause Alzheimer's disease. Heavy metals are metals that are found naturally in the environment, and become concentrated and potentially harmful due to a variety of human activities. They include mercury, copper, zinc, iron, and lead. We come into contact with these metals through food, air, and water. Those who work in the manufacturing industries may also be exposed to heavy metals occupationally. In small quantities, these metals are not dangerous, and some are even considered essential for good health. But in larger quantities, heavy metals have been linked to some chronic health conditions and diseases. In the past, it was hypothesized that lead (found in gasoline and paint manufactured before 1978), mercury (found in some dental fillings), and the nonessential metal aluminum (found in cookware, soda cans, and antiperspirants) might cause Alzheimer's. To date, however, researchers have found no clear association between these metals and AD.

There is some evidence that overexposure to copper (usually through food and water) may accelerate the progression from mild cognitive impairment (MCI) to dementia due to Alzheimer's disease.

It is believed that higher blood concentrations of free copper (copper that is not bound to proteins) may lead to either an increase in the accumulation of beta-amyloid protein or a decrease in the ability to process and clear those plaques. High free copper may also contribute to brain inflammation, which is a risk factor for AD.

At the same time, some studies indicate that copper may actually protect against AD. Further research is needed to clarify whether copper has a direct relationship with Alzheimer's disease.

Pesticide Exposure

There is some evidence that exposure to the pesticide DDT may increase the risk of AD in certain groups of people. One study found that in AD patients—especially AD patients who had the APOE4 genotype (see page 28)—the blood levels of DDE, a byproduct of DDT, were almost four times as high as those seen in people who did not have Alzheimer's. In addition, both DDT and DDE were found to increase the levels of beta-amyloid proteins in the brains of AD patients. While the agricultural use of DDT has been banned in most developed countries since the 1970s, other countries continue to use this substance, and you may come into contact with it through travel or the consumption of foods originating in these regions. Further research is necessary, but in the meantime, it may be sensible to limit exposure to DDT by avoiding nonorganic fruits and vegetables grown outside the United States, Canada, and other countries that have banned the use of this chemical.

Sleep Disorders

Mounting evidence suggests that sleep deprivation and a variety of sleep disorders (including sleep apnea) may contribute to cognitive decline and memory loss. It is not as certain if these problems contribute specifically to Alzheimer's disease. The importance of sleep for memory more generally is well established: Memories are consolidated (or strengthened) in the brain during sleep, so inadequate sleep may prevent memories from being formed and maintained. In addition, sleep is essential for allowing the brain to clear, or get rid of, amyloid deposits. Without enough sleep, the brain will accumulate more of these possibly harmful substances. Although recommendations vary, most research suggests that people should try to get seven to eight hours of sleep each night.

You may have heard of a substance called melatonin, which is a hormone produced by the brain that helps to regulate sleep-wake cycles. As we age, natural brain production of melatonin decreases, potentially making it difficult to fall asleep. In patients with AD, melatonin production is even further reduced. It remains unclear whether melatonin deficiencies or production shifts are associated with increased AD risk, or are rather a part of the disease process itself. Although there's no consensus yet, one study indicates that in people who are at risk for AD and have difficulty falling asleep, taking a melatonin supplement can improve sleep, cognitive function, and quality of life. Future research will help to clarify these points. (For information on using melatonin to treat insomnia, see page 207.)

Other Risk Factors

A number of other factors can also contribute to the risk of developing Alzheimer's disease. They include:

- Low educational attainment (no higher learning or participation in continuing education).

- Depression.

- Low thyroid function.

- Elevated levels of homocysteine (an inflammatory marker in the blood).

- Walking impairment.

- Chronic renal failure.

- Stress.

If you have—or suspect you have—any of these problems, talk to your doctor, who will best be able to advise you about steps you can take to improve your situation.

PROTECTIVE FACTORS

In contrast to risk factors, *protective factors* decrease the likelihood that a person will develop Alzheimer's disease. These factors not only shield the brain from damage, but may actually slow down brain aging. While this book focuses on one very powerful protective factor—diet—there are quite a few others, including:

- The APOE2 gene.

- Regular physical activity.

- Intellectual and social engagement.

- Greater educational or occupational attainment.

- Lifelong musical activity.

Several of the protective factors mentioned above work by contributing to something called cognitive reserve. Technically speaking, *cognitive reserve* represents the brain's resistance to damage and, thus, memory loss and cognitive decline. The concept arose from studies that attempted to explain why almost 40 percent of all people whose brains were found to bear the hallmarks of AD (beta-amyloid plaques and tau tangles) after death never showed any symptoms of dementia or decline beyond normal age-related cognitive impairment. Basically, cognitive reserve seems to be a sort of backup system for your brain, an extra store of cognitive ability, your mind's way of compensating for any brain damage or shrinkage that occurs in excess of the natural aging process. As a result, people with higher levels of cognitive reserve are less likely to develop Alzheimer's disease as they age. They also have better focus, memory, and overall thinking skills, and are able to maintain a higher level of cognitive function for longer periods later in life.

The development of this reserve begins at birth, accelerates during childhood and adolescence, and continues throughout young adulthood and middle age. Cognitive reserve may be determined in part by genetics, but scientists believe that life experiences are also contributing factors. Research suggests that people who challenge their minds—particularly earlier in life—tend to have higher levels of cognitive reserve. Learning more than one language, singing or playing a musical instrument, and having an extensive social network can all increase your cognitive reserve. Along similar lines, better cognitive reserve is associated with higher educational achievement (formal education beyond high school) and occupational attainment (reaching higher levels of success within one's job or field).

Scientists aren't sure how these behaviors protect your brain, but some believe that they improve cognitive performance by fostering new connections between your brain cells or by making existing networks of connections between brain cells more efficient or flexible. Whatever the case, it seems clear that an active mind is a mind that functions better and longer. (To learn about using physical activity, intellectual activity, and social engagement to help prevent Alzheimer's disease, see Chapter 7.)

THE DIAGNOSIS OF AD

There is no one test that can establish with 100-percent accuracy whether or not a living person has Alzheimer's disease. Currently, doctors can say with certainty that a patient has Alzheimer's disease only after he or she has died and an autopsy has confirmed the presence of the characteristic beta-amyloid plaques and tau tangles in the brain. However, recent advances in biomarker testing have improved the diagnostic process, enabling doctors to make better judgments. We hope that a time will come when early and correct diagnosis will be possible, but that moment is still a few years in the future.

If you suspect you might have MCI or AD, or if you believe you are at risk, a number of different physicians can evaluate you, including your primary care doctor (internist or family doctor), neurologist, geriatric psychiatrist (psychiatrist specializing in patients age sixty-five or older), or geriatrician (doctor specializing in the care of patients age sixty-five and over). We recommend seeing a doctor as soon as you start to experience symptoms, if not before. Anyone concerned about their risk should take measures to reduce it. The earlier the disease can be detected, the earlier it can be treated.

There are many different ways to diagnose the presence and stage of AD. Your doctor will probably use a variety of methods to arrive at a diagnosis. At the very least, your physician will take a comprehensive medical history and perform a thorough physical exam. Your doctor may also evaluate your cognitive skills with a basic test like the Mini-Mental Status Exam (MMSE). The MMSE is a thirty-point test that asks questions which evaluate a patient's orientation (sense of time and place), memory, attention, and language and visuospatial skills (such as the ability to process and copy an image by drawing it on paper).

Your doctor will also use blood tests and brain imaging to rule out other disorders that might cause dementia-like symptoms, such as a thyroid condition or the deficiency of a vitamin. Two brain imaging techniques—a computerized tomography (CT) scan or a magnetic resonance imaging (MRI) scan—may also be employed to determine whether the hippocampus, which is the brain's memory center, has shrunk. If you're seeing a neurologist, he or she will test your reflexes, muscle tone, coordination, and balance. Some doctors may also test how well your senses are functioning. Recent research has suggested that a decreased ability to identify certain familiar odors may be a very early symptom of the cognitive impairment of Alzheimer's disease. Similarly, cutting-edge eye- and skin-evaluating technology may be able to show a buildup of AD's characteristic beta-amyloid in the blood vessels of the retina, or in the skin. Because the research and technology behind these innovations are new, doctors do not routinely perform these tests.

In general, tests for biomarkers (see page 12) that indicate the presence of AD or other disorders which contribute to dementia are not commonly used by primary care physicians, but may be used at times by specialists, in specialized clinics and in research trials. This is because the technology is still new; more studies need to be performed to establish when it's most appropriate to use each test and on whom it should be used. Even when these tests are ordered, the results can be difficult to interpret due to the lack of scientific consensus about their meaning. For example, in 2012, the FDA approved a type of PET (positron emission tomography) scan that might be able to help diagnose specific types of dementia in patients with cognitive impairment. Unfortunately, a "positive" scan does not specifically establish the presence of AD, as opposed to another cognitive disorder. Finally, because their use has not become standardized, tests for biomarkers are quite costly, as they are not covered by insurance companies.

Right now, the new biomarker tests are reserved for occasions in which diagnostic uncertainty exists, such as when dementia symptoms are present in a young person without clear risk factors or a family history of AD. On these occasions, clinicians use a number of advanced techniques to look for AD hallmarks and biomarkers. PET imaging and brain spinal fluid (also called cerebrospinal fluid, or CSF) analysis can help detect the presence of beta-amyloid plaques, glucose metabolism issues, and other AD-associated brain changes, helping to more definitively establish a diagnosis.

Biomarker tests are very much a developing field, and one that holds a great deal of promise for the early detection of AD. New techniques and methods for detecting biomarkers—including brain imaging, brain wave scanning, sensitive neuropsychological testing, and sophisticated blood testing—are being cultivated all the time. Someday, a simple blood test may be able to tell us without a doubt whether a person has or will develop Alzheimer's. For now, more research needs to be done to clarify which biomarker tests for diagnosing AD are the most accurate, safe, and cost-effective.

It's important to note that genetic tests may accurately predict a future diagnosis of early-onset AD. As we've explained, early-onset AD is rare, and often caused by genetic factors. Genetic testing can help identify the specific mutations responsible, allowing these patients to enter research trials geared toward their genetic profiles. But the decision to have these tests is complex; your treating physician or a genetic counselor can help you determine whether these tests make sense for you. When it comes to determining the risk of late-onset AD, we generally discourage routine genetic testing. Finding out whether you have the APOE4 gene isn't always helpful; as we've explained, many people have the gene and never go on to develop AD. Moreover, testing for genes like APOE4 gives clinicians only one piece of a large and fairly complex picture of AD risk. While we do use genetic testing at the Alzheimer's Prevention Clinic, we do so to help personalize care recommendations and refine the data of patients who are participating in our research trials, not necessarily

Keeping an Eye on Alzheimer's Research Trials

As concern about Alzheimer's disease has grown over the years, the number of clinical research trials has increased. At any given time, hundreds of trials are being conducted to determine just which drugs, therapies, or interventions are most effective and safe for treating or preventing AD. Each trial has several different phases, and each phase helps researchers answer specific questions:

- *Phase I* evaluates a therapy's safety and side effects in a small group of subjects.

- *Phase II* evaluates a therapy's safety and side effects in a larger group (100 to 3,000 people).

- *Phase III* compares the therapy with standard treatment in a very large group of people. Safety and side effects are also monitored.

- *Phase IV* tracks the long-term safety, effectiveness, and optimal use of a drug that has been approved by the FDA.

It can take several years—on average, five to seven—for the results of a Phase III research trial to translate into meaningful therapies that can be prescribed by a physician. We have made tremendous progress in developing potential treatments, but more work has to be done before these therapies become available to the public.

Currently, AD researchers are investigating a large variety of treatments. Some studies explore drugs that specifically target amyloid and tau. Others determine whether medications used for other medical conditions could also be used to fight AD. And still other trials test nutritionally based therapies, from single nutrients to combination pills that incorporate a range of commonly available supplements. The trend in new research is to target patients in the earliest phases of AD—mostly, Stage 1 and Stage 2. After many trials, we have learned that the earlier in the disease process a potential therapy is tried, the more likely it is to benefit the patient.

to determine risk. Instead, we suggest that everyone focus on adopting a healthy lifestyle plan such as the one detailed in this book.

AD TREATMENT

At the present time, there is no cure for Alzheimer's disease. For patients who already have AD, treatment is geared toward managing symptoms and slowing the progression of the disorder. Medications, supplements, and other lifestyle changes are usually considered components of a comprehensive treatment program, and approaches vary according to both the doctor and the patient. We discuss dietary and lifestyle changes throughout the book, and in Chapter 7 (see page 200), we explain the various medications that are now in use to reduce AD symptoms and even stabilize cognitive function for a time.

While, as of yet, there is no one definitive and highly effective treatment for AD, scientists are learning more about the disease every day. Exciting clinical research trials are underway, and we are confident that better treatment options will become available in the years to come. If you would like to participate in one of the trials, we recommend visiting the National Institute on Aging's website on current research: http://www.nia.nih.gov/alzheimers/clinical-trials. Another good resource is www.AlzU.org/trials. There, you will find information on new trials near you.

THE PREVENTION OF AD

There is no guaranteed way to prevent the development of Alzheimer's disease. Instead, doctors primarily focus on minimizing the likelihood that their patients will develop the disease by managing or reducing the risk factors that make them more vulnerable. For example, your doctor may work on reducing your risk of heart disease by prescribing drugs or lifestyle changes that lower your cholesterol or blood pressure.

We believe that risk reduction is absolutely vital for anybody who is concerned about memory loss. This is in part because once a person actually has symptoms of AD, it is extremely difficult to regain memory function. While the diet we recommend in this book may help some people with AD stabilize or improve their memory, it is most optimal for individuals who have not yet been diagnosed with the disease. And because AD can develop in the brain decades before symptoms appear, we encourage everyone—not just those who have a higher risk of the disease—to adopt a brain-healthy diet.

As scientists continue to research the disease, more will become known about its root cause. And the more we learn about the origins of Alzheimer's disease, the better equipped we will be to prevent it.

CONCLUSION

In this chapter, we have given you a broad overview of Alzheimer's disease and shown you how our understanding of this condition has evolved over the years. Increasingly, scientists have come to believe that there is a great deal you can do to keep your mind clear and sharp for years to come.

Among other things, research increasingly suggests that diet may be a critical factor in both the treatment and the prevention of Alzheimer's. A good diet can help to stave off the disease in people who have not developed it and may slow the progression of the disease in people who have already been diagnosed. It is this fact that motivated us to write this book. In the next chapter, you'll learn why diet matters in the prevention and treatment of AD.

2.

———

Why Does Diet Matter?

In the decade that has passed since Alzheimer's disease was recognized as a major public health crisis, significant progress has been made in our understanding of the disease. Scientists have been able to home in on specific areas of research that seem to be especially significant for the future of AD prevention and treatment. And one of the most promising areas of their focus has been nutrition.

Recently, there has been an explosion of studies focusing on the effects of diet on brain function. Some evidence suggests that poor dietary and nutritional patterns may have contributed to the mounting prevalence of AD over the last twenty to thirty years. In part, scientists think that the Alzheimer's crisis is linked to rising rates of diet-related disorders such as diabetes. As we mentioned in Chapter 1, these conditions increase the risk of cardiovascular disease, which is itself a risk factor for AD. But newer research indicates that poor diet may not just be related to the risk of Alzheimer's—it may actually play a direct causal role in the development of the disease. Moreover, scientists now know that dietary modifications can be critical both to slowing the disease's progression and, potentially, to preventing it.

In this chapter, we will show you why diet has such a significant effect on Alzheimer's disease. First, we'll explain how the food you eat influences the way your brain works. Then you'll learn about two major nutrition-related conditions and how they may contribute to AD. Finally, we'll look into the newest research on diet and AD, introducing you to the concept of nutrigenomics, the field of study that examines the relationship between food intake and the expression of an individual's genes. This developing area of research gives us hope for the future, offering the potential for more targeted, individualized treatments for a number of different conditions, including Alzheimer's disease.

Much more remains to be learned about how diet can affect the brain. But the preliminary evidence makes it clear that nutrition is one of the most important factors in the management of Alzheimer's disease. Because this idea is so new, many people are not yet aware of it. We hope that someday, the importance of nutrition to cognitive health will be so well known and understood that people will take it for granted and will choose their foods with the intention of properly feeding their brain. In the meantime, we hope that the information in this chapter will spur you to make the best possible dietary choices for both brain function and overall health.

FEEDING YOUR BRAIN

As you know, the brain controls behavior. Among other things, it makes decisions about the food you eat. Until recently, however, the significant impact that this food had on brain function was largely overlooked.

On the most basic level, the food you eat provides fuel for your brain. Think of your brain as the finely tuned engine of a car. If you give your car low-quality fuel, the engine may break down before its time. But if you give your car high-quality fuel, the engine will work at peak performance for years to come.

Food influences the brain in different ways. Some nutrients affect the brain directly, because they are capable of crossing what scientists refer to as the blood-brain barrier. The *blood-brain barrier* is a complex network of special cells that separate the blood circulating throughout your body from the fluids that nourish and surround the brain. This barrier acts as a gatekeeper to your brain, keeping harmful chemicals out and allowing essential substances—like glucose, the brain's main source of fuel—to come in. Water, for example, is able to easily pass through this protective barrier, but harmful bacteria cannot.

At other times, food stimulates the release of certain chemicals that influence brain function—specifically, hormones and *neurotransmitters*, the chemicals that enable your brain cells to communicate. As one example, chocolate (especially dark chocolate) contains small amounts of both the neurotransmitter serotonin and its "building block" L-tryptophan, a substance that allows your brain to make more serotonin. Serotonin is a chemical responsible for happiness; it's the target of certain antidepressants, as higher levels of this neurotransmitter can make you feel better. By eating chocolate, you boost your brain's serotonin levels, and thus also boost your mood.

Because the kinds, quality, and quantity of the foods you eat can have such a significant effect on the way your brain works, it's important to regulate your diet to keep your mind operating at maximum capacity. To return to our original metaphor, over a lifetime, low-quality fuel can contribute to declining performance. The good news is that even for those who have not been consuming high-quality fuel, it's not too late to change! In fact, studies have shown that in just six weeks, a healthier diet can produce noticeable benefits to brain and body function. With the strategies we discuss in the rest of the book, you'll soon have your brain firing on all cylinders.

NUTRITION-RELATED CONDITIONS AND ALZHEIMER'S DISEASE

Over the last thirty years, the United States and other industrialized nations around the world have seen a tremendous increase in health disorders that are directly linked to poor diet and nutrition. Rates of obesity, diabetes, and *metabolic syndrome* (a cluster of conditions that increase the risk of heart disease and other disorders) have skyrocketed, due in no small part to the rapid growth of fast-food chains, larger portion sizes, and the availability of processed foods and foods with added sugars. People are eating more than they ever ate before, and they have dramatically increased their intake of sugar and fat while decreasing their intake of fruits and vegetables.

During the same period in which these nutrition-related disorders have increased, rates of Alzheimer's disease have also risen. This is no coincidence. For one thing, as we've mentioned, diabetes and metabolic syndrome are risk factors for heart disease, which is itself a risk factor for Alzheimer's. And diabetes has been independently linked to a higher likelihood of developing AD. In this section, we'll explore two of the most common problems and explain how they can contribute to cognitive dysfunction.

Excess Body Fat

The United States is suffering from an obesity epidemic. Over the last thirty-five years, obesity rates have doubled in the United States; by one estimate, the average American is more than twenty-six pounds heavier than he or she was in 1960. Today, more than one-third of all Americans, or about 79 million people, have obesity, which is characterized by a body mass index (BMI) of 30 or more. (See the inset on page 52). Only one country in the world—Mexico—has a higher rate of obesity.

How do we explain this national weight gain? Put simply, Americans are eating more than ever before. They're eating out more, too, spending more money on meals not made at home. This is a problem because over the years, portion sizes at restaurants, take-out establishments, and fast-food chains have increased considerably. The average restaurant meal today is about four times the size it was in the 1950s. At the same time, more food companies are offering larger sizes of popular items for relatively small increases in price. Why get thirty-two ounces of soda for a dollar when you can get sixty-four ounces for only a few cents more? Many of us are quick to jump on something that seems like a good deal.

But in the long run, the good deal turns bad. As a number of studies have shown, larger portion sizes encourage overeating. Worse still, because people have become accustomed to eating out, they've gotten used to these larger portion sizes. Nutritionists call this misperception *portion distortion*. As a result, even when Americans cook and eat at home, they consume much more than they need to maintain a healthy weight.

These changes in eating habits are at least partly responsible for the obesity crisis today. Obesity is a serious health condition, significantly increasing the risk of developing health conditions such as heart disease, stroke, diabetes, metabolic syndrome, gynecological problems, and certain kinds of cancer. It is also associated with a number of different brain-related issues. Research shows that those who have a higher BMI and waist-to hip ratio tend to see both lower total brain volume and greater shrinkage of the hippocampus (the brain's memory center) later in life. With fewer brain cells available, cognitive functioning suffers. A number of studies have reported an inverse relationship between body weight—particularly body fat—and memory function. In other words, having more body fat is associated with poorer memory. Higher "central adiposity"—basically, larger accumulations of subcutaneous and/or visceral fat in the abdominal area, or having a "beer belly"—is also associated with a greater risk of cognitive impairment.

As we mentioned in Chapter 1, obesity may be a specific risk factor for Alzheimer's disease. In one study, the findings of which were published in the journal *Current Alzheimer Research*, scientists followed ten thousand men and women ages forty to forty-five for an average of thirty-six years. The results indicated that individuals with obesity were more than three times as likely as normal-weight individuals to develop AD. Separate studies have shown that people who carry the so-called "fat gene"—the fat mass and obesity-associated (FTO) gene that is linked to a higher likelihood of becoming obese—have been shown to be more likely to develop Alzheimer's disease, especially when they also carry the APOE4 gene (see page 28). In addition, the FTO gene itself seems to be associated with reduced brain volume later in life. With that said, there is some conflicting evidence about whether obesity increases the risk of dementia. One study of nearly 2 million people in the United Kingdom showed that people who had clinically *severe* obesity (with a BMI over 40) actually had a 29-percent lower risk of dementia than did people of healthy weight. By contrast, people who were underweight (with a BMI under 18.5), had a risk of dementia that was 34-percent higher than that seen in healthy individuals. This study underscores the fact that the relationship between body weight and dementia is complex.

Scientists are not exactly sure how or why obesity increases a person's risk for developing AD. We do know that obesity leads to vascular disease, impaired insulin responsiveness, and defective glucose

Body Mass Index and Body Fat Percentage

Doctors use a standard of measurement called the *body mass index* (*BMI*) to determine whether a person is underweight, normal weight, overweight, or obese. In essence, the BMI compares a person's weight and height using a simple formula:

$$\text{BMI} = \frac{\text{weight in pounds} \times 703}{\text{height in inches}^2}$$

You can find automatic BMI calculators online—the websites for the Centers for Disease Control (CDC) and the National Heart, Lung, and Blood Institute both allow you to input your height and weight for instant results. (See page 233 of the Resources list for contact information.)

The table at right shows the four weight status categories in terms of calculated BMI ranges:

BMI does not take into consideration body fat percentage, which may be a more useful tool for establishing health risk than BMI alone. But as a marker of weight status, BMI is valuable in helping to predict

BMI	Category
Below 18.5	Underweight
18.5–24.9	Normal Weight
25.0–29.9	Overweight
30.0 & above	Obese

the likelihood that a person will develop a number of serious diseases and health conditions. People who are overweight or have obesity are considered to be at greater risk of developing hypertension, coronary heart disease, high cholesterol, diabetes, and at least ten types of cancer. In turn, these diseases may have long-term implications for your brain, increasing your risk of Alzheimer's disease and vascular dementia (dementia caused by impaired blood supply to the brain).

Another important measurement is *body composition analysis*, which looks at the proportion of fat and fat-free mass in the body. This measurement can be made using a variety of tools, including skin calipers, special scales, and other more sophisticated devices. Note that while scales that measure body weight and body fat are available for home use, they are not always accurate.

Body fat percentage can have a profound effect on an individual's health. Fat releases certain hormones that control body metabolism. One of the key fat cell hormones is *adiponectin,* which helps the body respond to insulin more effectively. Excess fat can lead to a decreased production of this key hormone, which can contribute to a host of conditions, such as metabolic dysfunction, cardiovascular disease, insulin resistance, and fatty liver disease. As you learned in Chapter 1, both cardiovascular disease and insulin resistance can have a negative impact on brain health.

A person's target body fat percentage will differ based on a variety of factors, such as gender and whether or not the individual is athletic. For example, according to the American Council on Exercise, an average adult male should have 18 to 24 percent body fat, and an average adult female should have 25 to 31 percent body fat. For athletic individuals, the targets are significantly lower—6 to 13 percent for athletic males and 14 to 20 percent for athletic females. As a person ages, these numbers generally rise to some degree.

In addition to body fat percentage, a person's body fat type and distribution are also critical to metabolism and overall health. Fat can be stored in a variety of places in the body. *Subcutaneous fat* is stored under the skin, *intramuscular fat* is stored in between muscles, and *visceral fat* is stored in and around the internal organs, such as the stomach and liver. This is a complicated topic, but in brief, visceral fat is far more dangerous than subcutaneous and intramuscular fat. Because visceral fat has been found to pump out certain harmful chemicals, too much visceral fat can lead to a number of negative health consequences, such as heart disease; high cholesterol; and, you guessed it, insulin resistance. Although there are precise tools available for researchers who want to calculate visceral fat, the simple measurement of waist circumference provides useful information regarding disease risk. For example, when a man has a large waist size over 40 inches in diameter, he is twelve times more likely than a man with a small waist size (29 to 34 inches) to develop diabetes, one of the more significant risk factors for AD. (See the inset on page 101 for information on approximating visceral fat.) The precise connection between body fat percentage, body fat distribution, and Alzheimer's disease is starting to become clearer, but more research is necessary to fully understand these complex relationships.

metabolism. Therefore, the negative effects of obesity may be due at least in part to diminished blood flow to the brain and/or poor brain energy metabolism. An in-depth discussion of these potential mechanisms is beyond the scope of this book, but the overall message is that obesity and memory loss are related, and a diet that helps prevent or lessen one is likely to have a positive effect on the other, as well.

Diabetes

As rates of obesity have increased in the United States, so, too, have rates of another nutrition-related condition that has its roots in higher weight: type 2 (formerly called "adult-onset") diabetes. *Type 2 diabetes* is a condition in which the body has a hard time processing glucose, a simple sugar that is the most basic form of energy required by all cells—including brain cells—in order to function. As a result, glucose builds up in the blood, potentially causing damage to the blood vessels, kidneys, eyes, and nerves over time.

These high glucose levels—a condition called *hyperglycemia*—are related to an underlying disorder called insulin resistance. *Insulin* is the hormone that helps your body regulate blood sugar, telling your cells to take in glucose. In *insulin resistance,* however, the body does not respond properly to insulin because it has become "resistant" to its effects. Accordingly, glucose stays in the bloodstream, causing hyperglycemia.

While scientists don't know the exact causes of insulin resistance, one potential contributor is a sustained diet high in carbohydrates, especially simple sugars. Most people know instinctively that too much sugar is "bad" and that it is related to obesity and diabetes. But few know why this is. To understand why a sugary diet can be dangerous, let's take a closer look at the insulin response.

Whenever you eat a meal, a certain amount of glucose is derived from your food and is released from your gastrointestinal tract into the bloodstream, through which it can travel to all the cells in your body. In response, your pancreas secretes a corresponding amount of insulin to help usher the glucose into your cells, where it's needed. Under ideal circumstances, the amount of insulin released is perfectly calibrated to the amount of glucose in your bloodstream. You'll have just the right volume of insulin to escort the glucose into your cells so that your body's *equilibrium*—chemical and physiological balance—is maintained.

But what happens if you eat a lot of sugary food? The carbohydrates break down into comparatively large amounts of glucose. And if you're eating carbohydrates with lots of simple sugars—like the kind that's added to coffee, tea, and baked goods—they break down into glucose very quickly. If you eat ten doughnuts in one sitting, your body will release an appropriately large volume of insulin to help process the glucose. If you keep overloading your system with doughnuts or other sugary items, however, your pancreas may eventually become overwhelmed by the need to keep up with the constant demand for insulin. Moreover, even if your body continues to produce the insulin required, the chances are good that your cells will become habituated to the hormone and stop responding, becoming insulin resistant. As a result, both the glucose and the insulin will build up in your bloodstream.

Insulin resistance is bad for your health in general: Unable to use the glucose in your bloodstream, your body stores a lot of this excess energy as fat. But studies increasingly show that insulin resistance is particularly bad for your brain. For one thing, high levels of insulin may contribute to the accumulation of beta-amyloid proteins, one of the hallmarks of AD (see page 10). Research indicates that insulin and beta-amyloid protein are both degraded (broken down) by the same enzyme, insulin-degrading enzyme (IDE). When the bloodstream is flooded with insulin, more IDE is needed to clear that insulin from your system. This may mean that there's less IDE available to break down and remove beta-amyloid proteins in the brain. Some researchers feel this leads to greater plaque growth and cognitive decline.

Scientists are still trying to work out the exact nature of the relationship between diabetes, insulin resistance, and Alzheimer's disease. But certain things are apparent. People who have diabetes are significantly more likely to develop dementia, and are more likely to develop Alzheimer's disease in particular. This may occur because of the reasons discussed above or because diabetes increases the risk of cardiovascular disease, which is itself a risk factor for AD. Diabetes may also increase the risk of developing mild cognitive impairment (see page 15). Studies suggest that even in people who do not have diabetes, high blood sugar levels—even borderline high blood sugar levels—are associated with accelerated cognitive decline. Research in this area is advancing rapidly, and one day, it may help define the optimal ranges of blood glucose.

Fortunately, there is much you can do to avoid developing type 2 diabetes, and in turn, Alzheimer's disease. Diet is the key here—and, as we've suggested, it is essential to choose carbohydrates with care. As you'll read in Chapter 3, not all carbs are created equal. There are different kinds of carbs, and you'll learn how to distinguish between them to avoid provoking the glucose overloads and insulin surges that can be so disastrous for your brain. Recent findings support the intake of healthier carbohydrates to assist cognitive function. In fact, a certain type of low-carb diet has been shown to improve memory performance in people with MCI.

In particular, we recommend limiting or cutting out the simple carbohydrates known as sugars. The United States has a major sugar problem. Our sugar obsession has progressed to the point where the average American consumes an astounding 130 pounds of sugar every year—mostly in the form of sugars added to processed and commercially manufactured food items. Why does this matter? Recent research suggests that sugar is an addictive substance on par with cocaine, if not even more deadly. Brain imaging studies have shown that eating sugary substances lights up pleasure centers in the brain more effectively than consuming fatty foods, alcohol, or drugs. As researchers like our colleague Eric Stice have demonstrated, sugar also excels at engaging the reward regions of the brain, driving compulsive eating and encouraging a vicious circle of sugar consumption.

The kicker is that the massive increases in sugar intake and our nation's addiction to sugar may have inadvertently been fueled by government programs designed to improve cardiac health. In the 1970s, dietary fat was thought to be the main cause of heart disease. To combat this problem, the government created regulations to lower the concentration of saturated fats in commercially available foods. But instead, the rate of heart disease increased!

Why? In an effort to make the new low-fat diet foods appealing, manufacturers replaced saturated fats with large quantities of sugar and/or high-fructose corn syrup. At the time, most people—even most scientists—believed that this was a fair trade. We now know, however, that sugar is converted into fat and stored in the body even more easily than dietary fat. And it is the sugar we consume that contributes not only to heart disease, but also to obesity, diabetes, Alzheimer's disease, and other forms of cognitive decline.

Overall, because of the knowledge we have today, we understand that a diet which is beneficial to people with diabetes is also beneficial to people who either have AD or are at risk for developing it. Limiting the intake of carbohydrates—especially sugars—may be the single most important component of any brain-healthy diet plan. (To learn more about carbohydrates, see page 68 of Chapter 3.)

NEW DIETARY CONCEPTS IN THE MANAGEMENT OF ALZHEIMER'S DISEASE

As scientists and medical professionals have come to accept the idea that a good diet can potentially prevent or slow the progression of Alzheimer's disease, researchers have begun to look at nutrition in new ways. In this section, we'll discuss three concepts that are on the cutting edge of AD research. While scientists are still working to learn more, caloric restriction, the use of ketones as brain fuel, nutrigenomics, and the gut microbiome may hold the keys to the future of AD prevention and treatment.

Caloric Restriction

The Japanese region of Okinawa has some of the longest-lived people on Earth. In 2000, life expectancy at birth was eighty-six years for Okinawan women and nearly seventy-eight for Okinawan men, with many surviving to one hundred and beyond. By current estimates, there are 35 centenarians (hundred-year-olds) in Okinawa in every 100,000 inhabitants. Moreover, mortality rates from the chronic diseases of aging—including cardiovascular disease, cancers, and dementias—are significantly lower there than anywhere else.

Looking for the keys to long life and healthy aging, in 1976, scientists began to study Okinawans. In the Okinawa Centenarian Study,

Dr. Bradley Willcox and his colleagues followed over 900 Okinawan centenarians and other Okinawans in their seventies, eighties, and nineties. They found that while genetics played a role in determining an Okinawan's lifespan, lifestyle factors like diet were also important. Compared with other Japanese, these older Okinawans ate less rice, grains, and other carbohydrates; they also ate more vegetables rich in antioxidants and other substances that are believed to slow aging. More important, however, the very old Okinawans had consistently consumed less food over their lifetimes, eating about 10 to 30 percent fewer calories than other Japanese people of similar ages and activity levels. On average, Okinawans consumed between 1,800 and 1,900 calories each day, and typically had BMIs between 18 and 22. By way of contrast, the average American eats between 1,800 and 2,600 calories and has a BMI of 26.5.

In essence, the Okinawans were practicing "caloric restriction"— a diet based on low calorie intake. Okinawans' caloric deficit arose in part due to agricultural and occupational necessities: Most Okinawans were farmers who expended a lot of energy over the course of their physically demanding day, and the local diet was built around vegetables like the sweet potato, which were low in calories but high in nutrients. At the same time, Okinawans had a cultural imperative to maintain caloric restriction. Many practiced a principle called *hara hachi bu*, a Japanese phrase that can be understood to mean, "Eat until you are 80 percent full."

The lesson we can take away from the Okinawan centenarians is that eating less may allow you to live longer, as well as to function at a higher level for longer. Unfortunately, the long-term effects of caloric restriction are largely unknown, due to the difficulty in getting people to comply with low-calorie diets for extended periods of time. Supporting studies, however, suggest that caloric restriction may be beneficial not only to healthy aging and longevity, but also to Alzheimer's disease and cognitive functioning. In 2012, researchers at the Mayo Clinic found that overeating could double the risk of memory loss. This study showed that eating more than 2,142 calories per day was associated with significantly increased odds of having moderate cognitive impairment. And the more a person ate, the greater the risk for developing MCI. In another study, researchers suggested that in people who are not overweight, caloric restriction leads to a lower BMI, lower body fat, lower cholesterol, significantly lower insulin levels, lower inflammatory markers, and lower blood pressure. Because caloric restriction thus lowers a person's risk for cardiovascular disease and helps to lower insulin levels, it also helps protect against AD. Research shows that caloric restriction may also have other benefits, such as helping cells function more optimally when under stress, decreasing cellular damage due to a condition called oxidative stress, reducing inflammation, and improving neurogenesis (the formation of brain cells), while helping to maintain cognitive abilities. Overall, when it comes to total calories, our recommendation is that less is more for optimal brain health.

Ketones—An Alternate Brain Fuel

Two different types of energy sources can fuel the brain. Similar to a hybrid car, which uses both gasoline and a rechargeable battery to power the engine, the brain can use both glucose and substances called *ketone bodies* or *ketones*, which are created when the body metabolizes (breaks down) fat. As an analogy, glucose is similar to gasoline, and ketone bodies are similar to a battery, since ketones are a cleaner-burning fuel.

There are two widely known ways to attempt to power the brain with ketone bodies. You can either make fairly significant changes in your dietary intake, or you can increase your intake of ketone body-producing substances.

The dietary pattern called the *ketogenic diet* requires a person to eat a high amount of fat and less than 20 or 30 grams of carbohydrates each day. This sends the individual into a state called *ketosis,* in which the body is deprived of the glucose it ordinarily uses as energy. Accordingly, it begins to manufacture an alternate energy source—ketone bodies—from the stored fat.

There is evidence to suggest that ketones may be a better energy source than glucose for AD patients. For one thing, an early characteristic of AD is an impaired ability to use glucose. When glucose is the only available energy source, this impairment can have profound effects on brain function, making the availability of an alternative fuel of vital importance. Also, very low-carbohydrate ketogenic diets can be beneficial in that they generally result in weight loss. Nevertheless, very low-carbohydrate ketogenic diets are, for the most part, rarely recommended. First, for certain individuals, prolonged ketosis may result in negative health consequences. For example, in certain diabetics—usually type 1, but sometimes type 2—very low-carbohydrate diets cause a dangerous condition called diabetic ketoacidosis. Additionally, to follow this type of diet, a person would require periodic laboratory assessments and need to be under the care of a treating physician and a dietitian. Finally, while a very low-carbohydrate diet may be an effective means of losing weight over the short term, it can prove difficult to maintain.

The second widely known way to power the brain with ketones is to increase the consumption of *medium-chain triglycerides* (MCTs), a type of saturated fat. In the next chapter, you'll learn that for the most part, saturated fats eaten in excess are bad for your health. But most saturated fat in the American diet is composed of long-chain fatty acids. Medium-chain fatty acids, on the other hand, have unique properties, and some scientists believe that they may be a sensible therapeutic option in the nutritional management of AD. MCTs occur naturally in certain foods and can be made even more potent nutritionally through the processing of naturally occurring coconut or palm oils. There are several different fatty acids classified as MCTs. While we don't yet know which types of MCTs may prove to be the most brain-healthy, we do know that these fats are digested and utilized differently from other fatty acids, resulting in the production of ketones even in the absence of carbohydrate restriction. Researchers are now studying caprylic triglyceride—a form of MCTs—to determine possible benefits for people who have been diagnosed with Stage 3 AD. It is thought that MCTs may be helpful for people who have certain genes, but may not be as helpful for individuals with a different set of genes. Ongoing clinical trials should bring welcome clarity to this exciting area of potential therapeutic intervention.

The Alzheimer's Prevention and Treatment (APT) Diet incorporates the brain-boosting benefits of ketones in a different way. We propose a sustainable program of dietary changes in which you reduce your carbohydrate consumption through more moderate measures than the ketogenic diet discussed earlier while also timing meals to facilitate the natural production of ketones by the body. Currently, the Institute of Medicine's Food and Nutrition Board sets the Recommended Daily Allowance (RDA) for minimum carbohydrate intake at 130 grams per day. Over the course of our nine-week diet plan, you will progressively decrease your carbohydrate intake until you're eating slightly less than the RDA, with a goal of about 100 to 120 grams each day. Moreover, five days a week, the carbs (as well as other nutrients) are eaten only within a continual period of eight to twelve hours—a period that ends with a twelve- to sixteen-hour overnight fast. This target allows you to eat many of the carbohydrates that you've always enjoyed, as long as you do so in small to moderate quantities. By including a certain amount of carbohydrates in your meals—mostly low-glycemic vegetables, fruits, and whole grains—you can easily maintain this diet for the rest of your life.

Be aware that this is not the very low-carbohydrate ketogenic diet discussed earlier. Instead of decreasing overall carbohydrate intake to 20 to 30 grams each day to induce ketosis, our diet plan more moderately reduces carbs, partly through a period of overnight carbohydrate restriction. After about twelve hours of restricted carb intake, the body starts to naturally produce ketone bodies to help fuel the brain. These carb-free periods also have the effect of reducing overall caloric intake and increasing insulin sensitivity and glucose metabolism.

We call this the "early-bird special" technique of brain-healthy eating. Available at some restaurants, the early-bird special is a discounted meal offered before traditional dinner hours, usually prior to 6:00 PM. It turns out that saving money isn't the only benefit associated with having an early evening meal! This strategy, pared with moderate carbohydrate restriction, can bring about a mild state of ketosis that provides the body with clean-burning, brain-healthy ketones. Of course, this means no late-night snacking between dinner and breakfast!

Nutrigenomics

Another dietary concept that may be critical to the future of AD therapy is *nutrigenomics,* a field of science that studies the relationship between food intake and genetics at a molecular level. This field has three primary areas of focus: how genetic variations determine an individual's response to specific nutrients and diets; how food influences genetic expression (the way a person's genes direct growth, behavior, and other actions); and how an individual's genes regulate nutritional requirements. AD researchers are most interested in the first concept—the idea that a person's genetics can shape the way he or she responds to a diet.

What nutrigenomics offers is the potential for more personalized disease treatment and prevention—not just for Alzheimer's disease, but for a number of different conditions. In time, nutrigenomics may help predict the therapies that will be most effective for each individual. As a result, doctors will be able to adapt their patients' diets and treatment protocols to their specific genetic profiles. Further study of genes that are associated with different clinical responses will also help people focus on which foods to avoid, and which to maximize, to optimally improve health.

When a person is evaluated at the Alzheimer's Prevention Clinic, several genetic tests are ordered to help make more targeted management decisions. It is important to note that these genetic tests are not ordered to help diagnose AD, but rather to aid direct treatment or prevention efforts. Dr. Isaacson looks for certain genes, and modifies his treatment according to their presence or absence. For example, B vitamins may be helpful for reducing the risk of cognitive decline in a subset of people with MCI—those who also have a high blood level of the amino acid homocysteine. People who decide to take B vitamins usually take the most common form of vitamin B_{12} (cyanocobalamin) and vitamin B_9 (folic acid). However, there are alternate chemical formulations of these vitamins that may be more appropriate for certain people. When people with a fairly common gene mutation called methylenetetrahydrofolate reductase (MTHFR) have an elevated homocysteine level despite taking the more common forms of B vitamins, a different form of B_{12} named methylcobalamin and a different form of B_9 called L-5-methyl-tetrahydrofolate may be more effective. Research is ongoing to help clarify these points. The alternate forms of these vitamins can usually be found in health food stores, although they're also available as a prescription medical food.

Similarly, a few studies have found that people who lacked the APOE4 gene have experienced cognitive benefits from supplementing their diet with certain omega-3 fatty acids and caprylic triglyceride. However, people who had the APOE4 gene did not experience this benefit. In the PREDIMED-NAVARRA study—a long-term study that examined the effect of the Mediterranean diet on cardiovascular disease risk—researchers found that people who had certain genes saw greater benefits from adopting a Mediterranean-style food plan. Specifically, individuals who had the "genetically favorable" profile of genes called CR1, CLU, and PICALM saw their cognitive performance improve much more significantly on the Mediterranean diet than did people with the same genetic profiles who were assigned a low-fat diet. While these genetic tests are usually ordered only in research settings, the findings underscore the effects of genes on an individual's response to specific dietary patterns.

Overall, personalized nutrition is an exciting and rapidly evolving area of research. While much work remains to be done to improve our understanding and use of nutrigenomics, doctors are beginning to apply the initial research results to patient care.

The Microbiome

Recently, a new area of investigation has focused on the *gut-brain axis*—the interaction between the gastrointestinal (GI) system and the nervous system, which includes the brain. Some researchers have referred to the gastrointestinal tract as a second brain, since it contains half a billion neurons that help control a variety of functions, including digestion, immune health, lipid metabolism, and even mood. In fact, most of your body's serotonin—the primary chemical that maintains mood balance and happiness—is produced by the GI system.

An important part of gut-brain axis research involves the *gut microbiome*—the population of microbes in the intestines. The gut houses trillions of bacteria; by some estimates, this mass of gut bacteria, or *microbiome,* weighs almost as much as the brain itself! These bacteria coexist with the body in a symbiotic relationship; humans need bacteria to survive, and the bacteria can't survive without a host. Scientists are beginning to speculate that the health of your gut microbes may affect brain function by impacting a myriad of body functions, including the absorption of energy from the foods you eat and the storage and expenditure of that energy. A healthy microbiome appears to contribute to normal weight, the normal use of glucose and insulin, and other mechanisms necessary for general well-being, including normal brain function. When the microbiome changes, these body functions are affected, as well.

One of the factors known to greatly affect the gut microbiome is diet. For instance, a diet high in processed food—in other words, the high-saturated fat, high-trans fat, high-sugar diet that is now so common—has been shown to adversely affect the gut microbes of mice within only twenty-four hours. Over time, this shift has been associated with an increase in body weight as well as chronic inflammation and the development of insulin resistance—all factors strongly associated with Alzheimer's disease.

Further research is needed to determine exactly how the microbiome can be adapted to improve brain health and prevent Alzheimer's disease. What is known now is that certain dietary components can contribute to the maintenance or restoration of normal gut bacteria. For instance, *probiotics*—live bacteria and yeast that are good for your health—can help create a balance between good and bad bacteria to keep your body working properly. Probiotics are supplied by yogurt that contains live and active cultures, by other fermented foods, and by supplements. Another dietary component that can help normalize the microbiome is *prebiotics,* which are certain nondigestible carbohydrates (fiber) that stimulate the growth of selective beneficial gut bacteria. Prebiotics occur naturally in a number of foods, including asparagus; garlic; onions; grapefruit; chickpeas; lentils; cashews and pistachios; and whole-grain wheat, oats, and barley.

The Alzheimer's Prevention and Treatment Diet helps to promote gut health by providing both probiotics and prebiotics through an emphasis on yogurt as a primary source of dairy; a plentiful intake of fruits and vegetables; and moderate amounts of whole wheat products, oats, barley, and legumes. Although there is surely more to be learned about this area of research, evidence now indicates that foods rich in pro- and prebiotics may have an appreciable impact on the prevention and treatment of AD.

CONCLUSION

Hopefully, this chapter has impressed upon you the importance of diet, not just for keeping or cultivating good brain function, but for maintaining your general health. So where do we go from here? What does the future hold for the study of diet and Alzheimer's disease? In the next decade, scientists will surely gain a better understanding of the specific dietary factors that contribute to the progression of Alzheimer's. As a result, they will continue to refine their strategies for AD prevention and treatment, paving the way for more effective care that is tailored to the genetic makeup of each individual.

Until then, the best thing you can do for your mind is to maintain a diet that is protective of the brain. To learn more about the components of a good diet, turn the page.

3.

The Elements
of Nutrition

In the previous chapter, we explained how food is fuel for the brain, and how the quality of that fuel can have a significant impact on brain and memory function. Now it's time to delve a little deeper into the question of the fuel itself. To understand the core principles of the Alzheimer's Prevention and Treatment Diet, it's important to learn a little about the elements of nutrition known as macronutrients.

Macronutrients are nutrients that the human body requires in relatively large amounts in order to grow, develop, and function. There are three main macronutrients: carbohydrates, proteins, and fats. Almost all human diets involve some combination of these three macronutrients in different ratios, and prior research has evaluated the effect that different amounts of these macronutrients have on human health.

In this chapter, we'll give you some basic information about carbohydrates, proteins, and fats. You'll read about how each macronutrient affects your cognitive function and overall well-being, and how you can distinguish between healthy and unhealthy types within each category. Because our nine-week program asks you to reduce your consumption of carbohydrates, we'll be paying special attention to that macronutrient, explaining how both the quantity and quality are critical to a brain-friendly diet.

The information in this chapter provides the scientific foundation for the dietary guidelines and strategies we will set forth in the next few chapters. By learning about macronutrients, you'll be better equipped to understand our recommendations, and you'll be more inclined to put this information into action.

CARBOHYDRATES

Carbohydrates are routinely the body's primary source of energy, breaking down into the sugar called glucose, which all cells need in order to function properly. Carbohydrates are produced by plants during the process of photosynthesis. Accordingly, any time you eat fruits, vegetables, legumes, grains, seeds, and products made from these plant-based food groups, you are eating carbohydrates— although plants can contain other macronutrients, as well. Trace amounts of carbohydrates can also be found in some types of meat, poultry, fish, dairy, and eggs. Carbohydrates form the basis of most diets around the world, traditionally accounting for at least half of all calories consumed, if not more.

If you're like most people, you grew up eating relatively high-carbohydrate diets when compared with the portion of your diet composed of proteins and fats. But are these diets good for your brain?

Minimizing the Quantity of Your Carbohydrates

As we explained in Chapter 2, the excessive consumption of carbohydrates can potentially contribute to a number of health conditions— including Alzheimer's disease—and simple sugars are especially problematic. Let's take a moment to review why this is so.

All carbohydrates break down into glucose during digestion. The glucose then enters the bloodstream and travels throughout the body. In response to these rising blood sugar levels, the pancreas secretes insulin, a special hormone that tells cells to absorb glucose so that they will have the energy they need. As the cells take in the glucose, blood levels of both glucose and insulin decrease.

Trouble arises when you eat more carbohydrates and sugars than you need. Your cells require only a certain amount of glucose for energy; the rest is stored as fat. Worse still, when you continually flood your system with glucose from carbohydrates, your body progressively becomes less capable of handling it. Your pancreas is overwhelmed and turns out large amounts of insulin in an attempt to clear the glucose out of your bloodstream. Over time, you can develop a condition called *insulin resistance:* Your cells simply stop responding to the insulin, refusing to take in more glucose. As a result, blood levels of glucose and insulin remain high. Between the insulin resistance, high blood sugar and insulin levels, and the greater accumulation of fat, excessive carbohydrate consumption can lead to obesity, diabetes, and metabolic syndrome, as well as cognitive dysfunction over time.

For these reasons, we recommend that most people reduce their carbohydrate intake. We want to be very clear here: Carbohydrates themselves are not necessarily bad! In fact, we all need carbohydrates in order to meet basic nutritional requirements. We do not promote the very low-carbohydrate diet known as the ketogenic diet, which was discussed in the previous chapter (see page 59). Rather, we advocate slowly and progressively decreasing your carbohydrate intake to 100 to 120 grams of "good" carbs each day. For most people, this is an attainable goal. Gradually restricting carbohydrate intake and limiting carb consumption to certain daytime hours helps reduce carbohydrate intake without creating a feeling of deprivation, while also improving insulin sensitivity and glucose metabolism.

In addition to paying attention to the amount of carbs you consume and the time of day you eat them, it is essential to be mindful of the *quality* of your carbs. When it comes to brain health, the kind of carbs you eat is of crucial importance. How can you tell the good carbs from the bad? That is the subject of our next discussion.

Maximizing the Quality of Your Carbs

As we explained earlier, not all carbohydrates are created equal. Some carbohydrates are better for you than others. Because the APT Diet places a special focus on regulating your carbohydrate intake, it's important to learn how to distinguish between the different types that are available to you.

Historically, carbohydrates have been classified according to their source, their chemical structure, and the ease or difficulty with which they are broken down into glucose. Under this classification system, there are two main types of carbohydrates: simple and complex. *Simple carbohydrates* have relatively uncomplicated chemical structures, being made of one or two sugar molecules. This causes them to break down into glucose very quickly when they're consumed. Simple carbohydrates—and their simple sugars—occur naturally in fruits, vegetables, and dairy products. They are found in relatively high amounts in processed or "refined" foods such as table sugar, brown sugar, corn syrup, fructose, and fruit juice concentrate; and in prepared foods such as sweetened beverages, baked goods, and candy.

By contrast, *complex carbohydrates* have more complicated chemical structures. They're made from chains of three or more simple sugar units that have been linked together. Because these carbohydrates are often rich in fiber, it takes the human body longer to digest and convert them into glucose. Complex carbohydrates tend to be thought of as starchy foods: whole grains and whole-grain products, legumes (beans, peas, and peanuts), and certain vegetables (such as potatoes and corn).

People are often advised to eat fewer simple carbohydrates and more complex carbohydrates. Although this is sensible advice, it's perhaps just a little bit simplistic. Terms such as "simple carbohydrates" and "complex carbohydrates" are now recognized as having relatively little nutritional or physiological significance. Instead of these terms, the World Health Organization suggests that we focus on the total carbohydrate content of food and on its glycemic index, the latter of which is relied on by many nutritionists to evaluate whether a carbohydrate is "good" or "bad."

The *glycemic index* (*GI*) was devised by Dr. David Jenkins in 1981. It is a system that indicates on a range of 1 to 100 how quickly a food elevates glucose levels in the blood. The higher the number, the more quickly the food triggers a rush of glucose. Foods with a high glycemic index—that is, foods with a rating of 70 to 100, such as a piece of white bread—cause your blood sugar levels to spike, or rise rapidly. Foods with a low glycemic index—foods with a rating of 55 or less, such as black beans—increase blood sugar levels much more slowly.

Whether or not you're conscious of it, you've probably experienced the effects of eating foods that rank high on the glycemic index. In the United States, many of us like to eat lunches that are based on high-glycemic carbs. We enjoy foods like bagels (with a GI of around 72) or French fries (with a GI of approximately 75) and feel momentarily energized as our blood glucose levels spike. But within an hour or two, we crash, feeling groggy and listless as our blood glucose levels rapidly decrease. Sound familiar?

Knowing what you now know about glucose levels and the insulin response, it should be clear that foods which rank high on the glycemic index tend to be less healthy, and foods that rank low on the glycemic index tend to be more healthy. And, in fact, studies have shown that diets rich in high-glycemic foods increase the risk of type 2 diabetes and heart disease. In view of this evidence, we usually recommend that people look for foods with a low glycemic index when choosing carbohydrates. Keep in mind that low-glycemic foods have benefits other than their effect on blood glucose levels. They are often richer in vitamins, minerals, and fiber. They also tend to have lower energy densities, containing fewer calories per serving. That means you can eat more of lower-glycemic foods without gaining weight. Consequently, many nutritionists recommend a low-GI diet to people who are overweight or have obesity.

For the most part, simple carbohydrates tend to have higher glycemic indices, and complex carbohydrates tend to have lower ones. This should make intuitive sense. Simple carbohydrates are easier to digest and break down, so the resulting glucose enters the bloodstream readily. Complex carbs take longer to digest, and thus release glucose into the bloodstream more gradually.

A variety of factors can affect a food's glycemic index. One of the most important factors is fiber content. Foods with higher fiber contents take longer to be digested and thus release glucose more slowly. Accordingly, they have lower glycemic indices. This means that while complex carbs like oatmeal are considered low-glycemic, some foods that are made up of simple carbs and sugars, but have plenty of fiber—foods like apples and tomatoes—are also low-glycemic. Fats and acids can also affect a food's glycemic index, making them more complicated to digest. For this reason, spaghetti with meatballs actually has a lower glycemic index than plain boiled spaghetti—the fats and acids in the meatballs and sauce make it harder for your gastrointestinal tract to extract the glucose. Other factors that contribute to a food's glycemic index include the level of refinement or processing (boiled whole wheat berries are lower on the glycemic index than breads made with whole-grain flour) and the ripeness of the fruit or vegetable (the riper the fruit, the more sugars it has, and the higher its glycemic index).

Although the GI system is helpful, it has its flaws, perhaps the most significant of which is that it ignores the amount of food consumed. GI values were determined by studies in which volunteers ate portions containing 50 carbohydrate grams of each test food. But in real life, people don't always eat a portion that provides 50 grams of carbs. That's why Harvard scientists introduced the concept of *glycemic load* (GL), which takes into account not only the glycemic index of a food but also the amount of carbohydrates provided by an *actual serving* of the food.

To better understand the difference between glycemic index and glycemic load, it's helpful to look at two foods, carrots and sweet potatoes, and see how their GIs contrast with their GLs. An amount of raw carrots that contains 50 carb grams—the standard quantity used to measure the glycemic index—elevates blood sugar and insulin levels much more quickly than an amount of sweet potatoes containing 50 grams of carbs. Carrots are thus rated as a high-glycemic-index food, and sweet potatoes are ranked somewhat lower. Of course, almost nobody eats this amount of raw carrots in one sitting—that's about three cups of carrots! A normal serving is much smaller and contains fewer grams of carbohydrates. Accordingly, the glycemic load of raw carrots is fairly low, signifying that it is, in fact, a healthy food to consume. Conversely, although sweet potatoes rank in the middle of the glycemic index, their glycemic load is high, due to the fact that an average serving of boiled sweet potatoes is comparatively larger than a serving of raw carrots, and thus contains more carbohydrates. This doesn't mean that you should avoid sweet potatoes altogether—these vegetables are high in many important vitamins and minerals. Rather, the high glycemic load tells you that if you choose to eat sweet potatoes, you should eat smaller amounts than you might ordinarily.

Scientists use a simple formula to calculate glycemic load:

$$\frac{\text{Glycemic index number} \times \text{number of carbohydrates (grams)}}{100} = \text{glycemic load}$$

Each unit in the glycemic load score represents the effect rendered by eating 1 gram of pure glucose. A glycemic load of 20 or more is said to be high; one between 11 and 19 is medium; and a GL of 10 or less is said to be low. Because a lower glycemic load indicates that a food has a lower total carbohydrate content and greater overall carbohydrate quality, it is considered to be better for you than a higher glycemic load.

Many nutrition experts feel that the glycemic load is a more useful tool than the glycemic index in determining the overall value of a given food. The glycemic load gives us more information about carbohydrate content, and also accounts for some anomalies in the glycemic index that would otherwise prevent you from eating some very healthy foods. If you were relying solely on the glycemic index to make your food choices, you'd have to avoid certain fruits and vegetables that actually provide valuable nutrients. You see, many fruits and vegetables rate high on the glycemic index, but are typically eaten in small servings that provide relatively few actual carbohydrates. Consequently, they are brain-healthy choices.

Time and time again, people believe that they are eating a healthy and balanced diet when they are actually having too many high-glycemic carbohydrates. To better understand why high-GI carbs are a problem, pretend that you are heating your house with a wood-burning stove, but that all you're tossing in is paper and kindling. The fuel burns quickly and intensely for a short period of time, and then burns out, leaving the house cold. That's what it's like to eat only high-glycemic foods. By contrast, eating low-glycemic foods is like building your fire with perfectly seasoned logs. Just as slow-burning logs keep the fire steady, low-GI foods regulate the amount of glucose that is released in your body, giving you a steadier supply of energy and avoiding the glucose spikes that can lead to AD-related health problems such as high blood sugar and insulin resistance.

Both the glycemic index and the glycemic load can help you determine the best carbs for your diet. Glycemic load is a bit more useful because it takes into account the glycemic index as well as portion size. The Alzheimer's Prevention and Treatment (APT) Diet is built on low-GI and low-GL foods, and also emphasizes a reduction

A Word About Gluten

In this chapter, we present a number of good reasons why you should limit your overall carbohydrate intake and carefully choose the food sources of those carbs you do eat. In recent years, scientists have begun to learn more about the effects of gluten—a protein found in many common carbohydrates—providing yet another reason to make smart carb choices.

About 1 in 141 Americans has *celiac disease,* a chronic digestive disorder in which the consumption of gluten triggers an intense immune reaction, causing inflammation and damage to the small intestine. Many more folks have a gluten sensitivity unrelated to celiac disease. People with either condition develop stomach pain, bloating, diarrhea, weakness, fatigue, and weight loss after eating carbohydrates that contain gluten—carbs that come from wheat, barley, or rye.

Currently, there is no evidence to support any direct relationship between Alzheimer's disease and celiac disease or gluten sensitivity. But these conditions may indirectly contribute to problems with thinking and memory. The inflammation caused by celiac disease and gluten sensitivity, for example, may extend to the brain, potentially damaging cells there and impairing cognitive function. Celiac disease and gluten sensitivity may also alter the expression of certain genes, with negative consequences for the brain. As a result, some preliminary studies indicate that people with gluten sensitivity or celiac disease may be at higher risk for a variety of neurologic disorders.

Some research has indicated that minimizing gluten intake could have potential benefits even for individuals who *don't* have celiac disease or gluten sensitivity. While further studies are needed to clarify what impact, if any, gluten has on brain health, it's worth noting that by limiting overall carbs, the APT Diet significantly reduces the dietary intake of gluten.

of the amount of carbohydrates. Combined, these strategies help avoid several health issues that are associated with AD.

There are a number of books and websites that provide exhaustive listings of the carb counts, glycemic index, and glycemic load of common foods. To find carbohydrate counts, we generally visit the USDA Supertracker website. To find glycemic index and glycemic load, we use the Mendosa.com Table of Glycemic Index and Glycemic Load. (See page 231 of the Resources list for more information on these websites.)

When you follow the Alzheimer's Prevention and Treatment Diet, will you have to look up the carbohydrate count, glycemic index, and glycemic load of each food? Since the APT Diet restricts carbohydrates, you will have to find and record carb counts—at least for the first few weeks of the diet. Eventually, you will know what the counts are for the foods you routinely eat and will spend less time looking them up. While it's important to understand what the GI and GL are, you do not have to research and record them, because in Chapter 5, we have provided handy lists of low-glycemic vegetables, fruits, and grains on which you should base your meals. (See page 124.) Moreover, the APT Diet (also presented in Chapter 5) automatically limits carbs by recommending moderate portion sizes of carb-rich foods. When you do want to look up the GI or GL of a food, though, the websites above will allow you to do so quickly and easily.

PROTEINS

Protein is a vital substance that all humans require to function properly. Every cell, tissue, and organ in your body contains protein. Without it, your body wouldn't be able to maintain and repair itself. Protein also facilitates many body processes. It is needed to make enzymes, which act as catalysts to bring about biochemical reactions; to make antibodies, which help fight infection; and to create DNA, which facilitates the building of all of the body's structures.

Proteins are made of building blocks called amino acids. Whenever you eat a protein, these amino acids are extracted during the process of digestion. There are twenty common amino acids, with each one performing a different function or functions within your body. Eleven of those twenty amino acids can be made by your body. Because they don't need to be derived from food, scientists call these amino acids *nonessential*. The other nine amino acids must be provided by the foods we eat. Accordingly, scientists call these amino acids *essential*, because they are essential to a healthy diet.

Amino acids play a key role in the brain because they are the building blocks of *neurotransmitters*, the chemical messengers that allow cells to communicate with one another. The ability of cells to talk to one another allows memories to be formed and stored. Thus, proteins are vital to the formation of memories. In addition, protein foods are often high in B vitamins, several of which appear to offer benefits to the brain.

Choosing Proteins

Because you will be reducing your carbohydrate intake on the Alzheimer's Prevention and Treatment Diet, the volume of protein you eat will increase somewhat. The Institute of Medicine recommends getting anywhere from 10 to 35 percent of your calories from protein per day. In a 2,000-calorie diet, that is equal to 50 to 175 grams of protein, which is a wide range. In the APT Diet, you will find that you are at the higher end of this range for protein. Everyone— whether or not they're following the APT Diet—should eat *at least* 1 gram of protein for every 2 pounds of body weight. This means that a 180-pound man will need at least 90 grams of protein, while a 110- pound woman will require at least 55 grams. To give you a frame of reference, a 3-ounce serving of chicken—a serving that's about the size of a deck of cards—contains about 20 grams of protein. Note that these are *minimum* recommendations. Exceeding these amounts of protein, as we do in our diet, is generally safe for individuals who do not have renal (kidney) disease or a family history of renal disease. Individuals who have or are at risk for renal disease should consult their physician regarding protein intake.

In the APT Diet, a large part of each meal will come from proteins that are complete or near-complete. This means that, alone or in combination, they will supply the body with all nine of the essential amino acids that are necessary for healthy functioning. Further, the diet emphasizes lean proteins, which do not supply a large amount of saturated fat. For example, white meat chicken is a more sensible choice than fattier dark meat chicken. Similarly, eating a fatty cut of red meat, such as prime ribs, should be avoided, but a leaner cut of grass-fed beef, like a filet, is fine on occasion. (Based on the recommendations of the World Health Organization, we suggest no more than one serving a week of red meat, and no processsed meats.) Finally, avoid protein that is imbedded in carbohydrates. For example, 1 cup of pasta provides 14 grams of (incomplete) protein, but also delivers a whopping 78 grams of carbs! Since the APT Diet limits carbs, pasta is not a good choice.

We refer to foods that deliver complete or near complete protein, but provide little or no saturated fat or carbohydrates, as *high-quality protein*. The primary sources of high-quality animal proteins that we suggest for nonvegetarians include poultry (as many times a week as you like, as long as you remain within any calorie budget your doctor might provide); omega-3-rich fish (at least twice per week); eggs (four to eight per week); and lean beef and pork (no more than once a week). When you're buying lean beef or pork, choose grass-fed, since it will have higher levels of brain-healthy omega-3 fatty acids. (You'll learn more about these fats later in the chapter.) When you're buying fish, choose wild-caught over farm-raised, as farmed fish tends to have higher levels of pesticides, toxins, and other potentially cancer-causing compounds.

Dairy products can also be a good source of protein, but much of the research suggests that these products should be eaten in moderation rather than high amounts. To further protect your health, we recommend limiting butter and cream to one tablespoon a week, and reducing full-fat dairy products to one or less serving a day, as these products are higher in saturated fat. It's important to also consider the source of the dairy. Butter, milk, and cream that come from grass-fed cows are believed to have a higher content of brain-healthy nutrients, including omega-3 fats. For this reason, you want to look for grass-fed low- or no-fat options. Also check the nutritional information on the package to make sure that the company isn't substituting sugar or sodium for the fat it's removing. As you've learned, sugar is just as dangerous as fat when it comes to your health—if not more dangerous!

If you are a vegetarian, and particularly if you are a vegan, getting enough protein may be challenging. However, plant-based protein is widely available and delicious, although most plant sources provide only *some* (not all) of the essential amino acids. Nuts, legumes (beans), and seeds like hemp and chia are excellent sources of protein and are suggested as part of a brain-healthy diet. Whole grains in moderation (one to three servings per day) are another good option. A variety of vegetables—sun-dried tomatoes, spinach, broccoli, kale, peas, onions, and garlic, for instance—are also fairly high in

---

Choosing Protein Powders

As you now know, the Alzheimer's Prevention and Treatment Diet emphasizes a food plan that's plentiful in high-quality proteins and relatively low in carbohydrates. But some people—especially vegetarians—may find it difficult to get the amount of healthful protein they need solely through the foods they eat. If this is true for you, we recommend supplementing your diet with protein powder.

When it comes to buying protein powders, we find that whey, soy, or egg-white proteins are all reasonable choices. Of these, we particularly recommend whey protein. This product has the highest *net protein utilization ratio*, meaning that with respect to the total volume of amino acids it supplies, a relatively high number can be converted into protein in the body. Whey protein also has the highest *protein efficiency ratio,* which signifies that your body can digest and use it more quickly than it can soy or egg-white protein. Because whey protein is the form of powdered protein that is most easily and efficiently used by the body, it is the best option for most people who want to protect their brain health through a higher-protein diet.

Shakes made with protein powder are not only a good way to add protein to the diet, but also perfect for making a fast and healthy meal replacement. (See page 148 for more on meal replacements.) And when unintended weight loss is a problem, high-protein shakes can be a good source of extra calories. (See page 197.)

---

protein. Finally, all-natural soy products such as edamame (young soybeans) and tofu are good choices for lean and *complete* proteins. Soy foods can be consumed several times each week, and when combined with vegetables, grains, nuts, and legumes, they make it possible to maintain a balanced diet that provides adequate protein for brain health. Vegetarians not able to derive sufficient amounts of protein from food should consider supplementing their diet with a protein shake, ideally using a protein powder that contains whey protein isolates. (See the inset on page 78.)

FATS

Contrary to what you might have learned growing up, fats are an integral part of any healthy diet. We all need fat in order to function. Fats help maintain your skin and hair and allow you to absorb certain vitamins. Certain fats actually help clear cholesterol—especially the "bad" low-density lipoprotein (LDL) cholesterol—from the body. About 60 percent of brain matter consists of fats. And, as you will discover in the pages that follow, certain fatty acids are so beneficial to memory function that we recommend consuming relatively large amounts of them, and we encourage people who can't get enough of these substances through food—especially those who have insufficient levels in their blood—to talk with their doctor about taking fatty acid supplements. Like so many other areas of Alzheimer's research, this is a growing field in which new information on preventing and fighting AD is always becoming available. So far, it's clear that fats can make a difference in brain health.

Just as there are good carbs and bad carbs, there are good fats and bad fats. In this instance, the "goodness" of any particular fat partly depends on its effect on your cholesterol levels. Cholesterol isn't bad in and of itself—your body needs a certain amount of this substance in order to make several important compounds, including vitamin D, estrogen, and testosterone. But high cholesterol in the blood—particularly a high ratio of "bad" low-density lipoprotein (LDL) cholesterol in proportion to "good" high-density lipoprotein (HDL) cholesterol—is considered a major risk factor for cardiovascular disease, which is itself a major risk factor for AD and other dementias. In fact, a good deal of evidence supports the theory that elevated levels of blood cholesterol are associated with the development of Alzheimer's disease. Damaging fats like trans fats increase your LDL cholesterol levels and decrease your HDL cholesterol levels, as well.

Below, we'll first discuss the fats that should be avoided or eaten in only limited quantities. We'll then look at fats that are known to improve cardiovascular health and, just as important, that show potential in the fight against AD.

Steering Clear of Trans Fats

Trans fats are the worst of all the fats, linked to obesity, heart disease, accelerated aging, and cancer. These fats increase LDL cholesterol, decrease HDL cholesterol, and are difficult for the body to break down. Not surprisingly, studies have shown that diets high in trans fats are associated with Alzheimer's disease.

There are two kinds of trans fats: naturally occurring trans fats and artificial trans fats. The two kinds are considered to be equally unhealthy. Naturally occurring trans fats are found in certain meats and dairy products, although in small amounts. Artificial trans fats are manufactured in an industrial process that adds hydrogen to liquid vegetable oil. The result is something called *partially hydrogenated oil,* which is solid at room temperature and shelf-stable. This means that it can be kept and used easily and for a much longer time than liquid oils. For this reason, many restaurants and fast-food chains use partially hydrogenated oil to deep-fry foods. Trans fats can also be found in popular commercially prepared foods, including baked goods (cakes, cookies, etc.), snacks (potato, tortilla, and corn chips), and stick margarines. About half of the trans fats we consume are created during food processing.

In recent years, one state (California), several counties (Montgomery County, Maryland; Nassau and Albany Counties, New York; and King County, Washington), and a number of cities (New York City, Philadelphia, and Tiburon, California) have banned the use of trans fats in restaurants. In 2013, the Food and Drug Administration announced that its panel of scientific experts no longer considers partially hydrogenated oils to be "Generally Recognized as Safe," or

GRAS. This is a groundbreaking ruling, because under the law, foods containing additives that are not GRAS cannot be sold. In 2015, the FDA took a step toward eliminating most trans fats from food by giving manufacturers three years to remove partially hydrogenated oils from their products.

Because it will take time for a policy change to be implemented, it's important that you be aware of the trans fats that are still present in many of the foods currently available to you. When purchasing any item, look carefully at the ingredients and nutritional information. Technically, as long as a food contains less than half a gram of trans fats, the label can still claim that it has zero grams of trans fat. But even if it looks like there are zero grams of trans fat, the ingredient list may tell you otherwise. If you see the words "partially hydrogenated" anywhere on that list, you will know there are at least small amounts of trans fats in the item you have in your hand. For the APT Diet, we recommend that you do everything you can to eliminate trans fats from your diet, or that you at least reduce your consumption of these harmful substances.

Limiting Saturated Fats

Saturated fats received their name because they have the maximum possible number of hydrogen atoms attached to each carbon atom, and are therefore "saturated" with hydrogen atoms. For the most part, when eaten in excess, these fats are bad for your health. This may be especially true for certain people, so you are encouraged to talk to your treating physician about this component of your diet.

Saturated fat is primarily found in meat, poultry, and dairy products, although it also occurs in some plant-based products, including palm oil and coconut oil. As discussed in Chapter 2 (see page 60), certain types of saturated fats (MCTs) are considered brain-healthy, but depending on the source and the type, other forms are thought to be damaging.

Strong evidence indicates that diets high in saturated fats are bad for your brain. In one major study, researchers found that people who eat foods rich in these fats may be as much as 2.4 times more likely to develop Alzheimer's disease than people who eat a more balanced diet. Some researchers believe that saturated fat is harmful because it may increase blood levels of cholesterol. It has also been observed that a diet high in saturated fat reduces the body's ability to clear beta-amyloid plaques, one of the hallmarks of AD.

The complicating factor here is that science is continually evolving, and the jury is still out regarding the exact amount and type of saturated fat that can be included in a brain-healthy diet. As we briefly discussed earlier, when it comes to certain meats (beef and pork) and dairy products, the type of diet that was given to the animal may be a key consideration when judging the positive or negative impact of these foods on the brain. That is why we recommend choosing grass-fed beef, pork, and dairy products. Another factor that must be considered is that certain people, depending on their genetic makeup, may be able to tolerate or even benefit from certain amounts of saturated fat, while others may experience a more negative impact from these fats over time. A further complication is that while experts long believed that there was a clear association between saturated fat intake and important risk factors for AD, like cardiovascular disease and diabetes, some recent studies have *not* found such a connection. Although more research is needed to explain these results, due to their intricacy, these studies are not likely to be carried out soon.

Based on the best evidence to date, the APT Diet limits saturated fats to approximately 10 percent of your dietary intake, which is in line with the most recent United States guidelines. We also recommend the regular monitoring of vascular risk factors (such as cholesterol levels) by your physician, seeing a nutritionist if advised, and modifying saturated fat intake as needed.

Benefiting from Unsaturated Fats

Now that we have discussed the types of dietary fat that have been implicated in the development of Alzheimer's disease, it's time to discuss unsaturated fats—a group of fats that has been found to support health in many ways. There are two main kinds of unsaturated fats: monounsaturated and polyunsaturated. Both are considered beneficial, although there are important differences even between these healthy fats.

Monounsaturated fats—so-called because each fat molecule has one unsaturated carbon bond—improve blood cholesterol levels, and for that reason, eating foods that are rich in monounsaturated fats can help reduce your risk of heart disease. And the benefits don't end there. Monounsaturated fats can also improve insulin levels and blood sugar control, reducing your risk of insulin resistance and diabetes—both of which are AD risk factors. You can find monounsaturated fats in avocados and in many nuts and seeds, including almonds, hazelnuts, pecans, and pumpkin and sesame seeds. They are also abundant in olive oil, which is the primary oil recommended for use on the APT Diet.

Polyunsaturated fats received their name because each molecule of fat contains more than one unsaturated carbon bond. As we have already stated, these fats are known to provide substantial health benefits. This is true in part because this category of fats includes omega-3 and omega-6 fatty acids—two essential fats that your body needs but is unable to manufacture on its own. Both of these fats are necessary for a number of body processes, including healthy brain development and function. But there is a truly significant difference between these fatty acids that has a tremendous impact on health: Omega-3s have an anti-inflammatory effect, while omega-6s have a pro-inflammatory effect. This does not mean that omega-6s are bad; after all, short-term inflammation is necessary for survival. (If you cut yourself, for example, the inflammatory response is necessary to stop the bleeding and start the healing process.) But when inflammation is fueled to the point that it becomes chronic, it promotes the development of a number of serious conditions, including Alzheimer's disease. That's why omega-3s and omega-6s have to be present in the diet in proper balance.

Studies have shown that an omega-6 to omega-3 ratio of 4 to 1 is a reasonable target, yet for some people, an even lower ratio of 3 to 1 may be better. Unfortunately, modern diets tend to have omega-6 to omega-3 ratios closer to 15 to 1. In other words, our diets generally provide way too much pro-inflammatory omega-6 fatty acids and too little anti-inflammatory omega-3 fatty acids.

How can you turn your diet around so that you take in less omega-6s and more omega-3s? One important step you can take is to reduce the consumption of vegetable oils high in omega-6s—including corn oil, sunflower oil, soybean oil, and cottonseed oil—as well as the salad dressings and other processed foods that contain them. Another important step is to optimize your consumption of omega-3s by following a diet that emphasizes fruits and vegetables, whole grains, fatty fish, and olive oil. As you will learn in Chapter 5, the Alzheimer's Prevention and Treatment Diet fits the bill by including an abundance of omega-3-rich foods and minimizing the consumption of processed foods.

While, as a general rule, it is best to consume these nutrients directly from food sources, as just described, a variety of studies have shown that omega-3 fatty acid supplements may have a beneficial effect on the brain. In our work at the Alzheimer's Prevention Clinic, we emphasize the consumption of the omega-3 fatty acids docosahexaenoic acid (DHA) and, in somewhat lesser amounts, eicosapentaenoic acid (EPA). Several studies have shown the potential benefit of these omega-3s whether supplied via food, such as fish that's high in fatty acids, or supplied through nutritional supplements in capsule or liquid form. One study—the Memory Improvement with Docosahexaenoic Acid Study (MIDAS)—showed that adults over the age of fifty-five with age-related cognitive decline demonstrated improvements in memory skills after taking 900 milligrams of algae-based supplements each day. (For more information on omega-3 fatty acid studies, see page 171.) It should also be noted that DHA is known to be essential for the growth and development of the brain in infants and for the maintenance of normal brain function in adults. In other words, DHA is a vital nutrient for the brain. That being said, it's important to add that we still have a great deal to learn about these nutrients. Some studies have found omega-3s to be helpful in the *prevention* of AD, but not in the *treatment* of existing AD. Other studies have found that omega-3s work better in some patients than in others.

Despite some conflicting data, at this point, studies suggest that diets containing healthy levels of unsaturated fats may help protect against Alzheimer's disease. For that reason, as already discussed, the Alzheimer's Prevention and Treatment Diet recommends foods that are rich in the most beneficial of these fats. In Chapter 6, we also discuss the use of omega-3 supplements. (See page 171.)

Keep in mind that while healthier fats appear to be a valuable tool in the fight against Alzheimer's disease, all fats, good and bad, are calorically dense, containing 9 calories per gram, while carbohydrates and proteins provide only 4 calories per gram. This is why, when you add good fats to your diet, you need to avoid the overconsumption of this macronutrient.

CONCLUSION

Our understanding of the dietary influences on Alzheimer's disease is still evolving. Nevertheless, as this chapter has shown, studies have already told us a great deal about the way different macronutrients—the basic elements of nutrition that include carbohydrates, protein, and fat—affect your brain's capacity to function properly. In Chapter 5, you'll learn how we apply the principles reviewed in this chapter to the Alzheimer's Prevention and Treatment Diet. But in the next chapter, we will review other brain-healthy diets—diets that, in many cases, have been the subject of research—with the goal of helping you better understand how the APT Diet combines proven dietary strategies to create a unique and effective eating plan.

4.

Diets That Improve Brain Health

Over the last decade, the interest in utilizing nutrition to enhance brain health and to avoid or manage neurological disorders has vastly increased. With the goal of identifying or developing a diet that can prevent cognitive decline, studies have looked at the effect of nutrition on specific cognitive functions such as executive function (the set of skills that enable you to get things done) and memory, as well as on existing disorders such as mild cognitive impairment (MCI). In some cases, studies have also tracked health conditions such as insulin resistance and inflammation, which have been found to be associated with Alzheimer's disease (AD). As you might suspect, any diet that promotes sound cardiovascular health, reduces insulin resistance, facilitates weight loss, and otherwise supports physical well-being has also been found to have a positive effect on brain health and performance.

This chapter looks at various diets that have been studied for their potential in preventing, slowing, or managing AD. For each diet, we first describe the eating plan, and then briefly review the studies that have been conducted on its brain-healthy effects. The chapter ends by examining the Alzheimer's Prevention and Treatment (APT) Diet.

Before we explore the individual diets, it's important to explain that nutrition can be investigated at several different levels. For years, researchers focused mostly on the effects of individual nutrients (such as vitamin E) or groups of nutrients (such as omega-3 fatty acids or antioxidants) on health. More recently, studies have focused on what is called a *dietary pattern*—a specific style of eating that is usually referred to simply as a *diet*. The studies we cite in this chapter focus on dietary patterns—eating plans that are believed to foster better brain health through combinations of high-nutrient foods; through the restriction of calories; and/or through the restriction of specific macronutrients, such as carbohydrates.

THE MEDITERRANEAN-STYLE DIET

In the mid-1900s, researchers—chief among them, biologist and physiologist Ancel Keys—observed that the traditional diet of the Mediterranean region, especially southern Italy and Greece, was associated with many health benefits, including a reduced risk of heart disease, a reduced risk of cancer, and a longer, healthier life. Later studies showed that it reduces inflammation, oxidative stress, and insulin levels.

What is a Mediterranean diet? It includes plentiful amounts of fresh, whole plant-based foods, including vegetables, whole grains, legumes, and nuts as the primary sources of carbohydrates. It uses heart-healthy olive oil instead of saturated fats like butter as the primary source of fat. And it includes low to moderate amounts of fish and lean poultry (at least twice per week) as the primary source of protein, and limits red meat to no more than a few times a month. It also includes moderate amounts of low-fat yogurt and milk, and low to moderate amounts of red wine. Perhaps as much a lifestyle as a food plan, the Mediterranean diet also includes regular physical activity.

Based on studies, the Mediterranean diet is considered by some experts to be an excellent method for reducing the risk of Alzheimer's disease. By one estimate, this diet can decrease AD risk by as much as 40 percent in older patients. The more strictly patients adhere to the diet, the more dramatically their risk is reduced. The Mediterranean eating plan is also believed to significantly reduce both the risk of developing mild cognitive impairment and the risk of developing AD in patients who already have MCI.

Why Aren't There More Head-to-Head Comparisons of Diets?

Aside from the Ros trial discussed on page 90, there here have been relatively few studies that have directly compared the effects of different diets on Alzheimer's disease. One important study, conducted by Jennifer L. Bayer-Carter and colleagues in Seattle, randomly assigned both cognitively healthy adults and adults with amnestic mild cognitive impairment (aMCI)—memory problems that may be a precursor to Alzheimer's—to one of two diets. One group followed a high-saturated fat/high-glycemic index (GI) diet, while another followed a low-saturated fat/low-glycemic index diet. MCI patients who adhered to a low-saturated fat/low-GI diet demonstrated a significant improvement in memory performance when compared with patients who followed a higher-fat, high-GI diet.

In an ideal world, there would be many more of these head-to-head studies, but unfortunately, that is not the case. Randomized studies of diet are quite complex to perform for a variety of reasons, including the difficulty involved in getting human subjects to adhere to a diet over time; the difficulty of determining which dietary strategy (limiting carbohydrates, limiting saturated fat, etc.) caused the change; and the difficulty in acquiring funding for nutrition-focused studies in a society that is more inclined to finance studies of pharmaceutical agents. Fortunately, literally hundreds of other studies have helped fill information gaps and point the way toward brain-healthy nutrition.

At the Alzheimer's Prevention Clinic and at partner institutions throughout the world, we strive to learn more about the best nutrition for cognitive health through both head-to-head studies and the close observation of patients who seek care in the clinic. We hope and expect that over time, research will yield new and better answers for everyone who wants to improve brain health and avoid, slow, or even reverse cognitive decline.

The Mediterranean diet may even affect brain function directly. Some evidence suggests that the diet may reduce the buildup of amyloid plaques in the brain. Perhaps as a result, research indicates that this eating plan can actually improve memory function and cognitive performance in both patients with MCI and patients with AD. It may also slow cognitive decline.

Although the Mediterranean diet has a number of components that help make it beneficial to your health, scientists often single out the types of fats it supplies for special notice. The Mediterranean diet is not a low-fat diet; as much as 30 percent of all calories consumed on the diet come from fat. In particular, those calories come from unsaturated fats—the polyunsaturated fats derived from nuts and fish, and, perhaps more important, the monounsaturated fat found in olive oil. Several studies have shown that this high intake of olive oil and other unsaturated fats may contribute heavily to the Mediterranean diet's ability to protect against Alzheimer's disease and other forms of cognitive decline.

A study that was published in 2015 in *JAMA Internal Medicine* by researcher Dr. Emilio Ros and colleagues provides the highest-quality evidence that this eating plan prevents cognitive decline. A total of 447 cognitively healthy volunteers were randomly divided into three groups, each of which was assigned a specific diet and was then monitored over a four-year period. One group followed the Mediterranean diet supplemented by a liter of extra virgin olive oil per week. Another group followed the Mediterranean diet supplemented with 30 grams per day of mixed nuts, including walnuts, hazelnuts, and almonds. And the third group followed a low-fat diet. Compared with the low-fat diet group, cognitive function in the areas of attention and executive function were better in the Mediterranean diet plus olive oil group, and memory function was better in the Mediterranean diet plus nuts group.

THE KETOGENIC DIET

Devised in the 1920s, originally as a treatment for epilepsy, a ketogenic diet—of which there are several versions—is a high-fat, moderate-protein, low-carbohydrate diet. The goal of the diet is to change the way in which the body is fueled. In Chapters 2 and 3, you learned that after you consume carbohydrates, they are broken down into glucose, which—under normal circumstances—is transported to and absorbed by the cells, where it is used to fuel the body. By reducing the amount of carbohydrates consumed to less than 20 to 30 grams of carbohydrates each day, a ketogenic diet creates a metabolic state called *ketosis,* in which, instead of burning glucose for fuel, the body burns fragments of fats called ketones.

In 2012, Dr. Robert Krikorian and colleagues aimed to determine how ketosis would affect people with mild cognitive impairment (MCI). Patients with MCI were randomly separated into two groups. One group was given a high-carbohydrate diet, and the other, a very-low-carbohydrate diet. After six weeks, the patients who had followed the low-carbohydrate diet demonstrated improved verbal memory performance and also experienced weight loss, decreased waist circumference, decreased blood sugar levels, and decreased fasting insulin. This study highlights a number of key points. First, the beneficial effects of diet were seen in a rather short period of time—just six weeks. Second, in addition to improvements in cognitive function, benefits were seen in a number of vital areas related to brain and body metabolism.

While scientists can only speculate about the exact mechanism through which a ketogenic diet can improve brain function, we do know that people with Alzheimer's have a higher prevalence of insulin resistance, which, over time, is believed to interfere with brain function and also act independently to promote harmful changes in the AD brain. As discussed in Chapter 2, we believe that ketones are a more efficient energy source for the brain than glucose, and that they help improve the function of the *mitochondria*—the "batteries" of the brain cells. That's why our nine-week Alzheimer's Prevention and Treatment Diet incorporates these concepts in an effort to optimize brain fuel metabolism and help protect against the progression of AD.

THE MIND DIET

In 2015, Dr. Martha Claire Morris and colleagues at the Rush University Medical Center in Chicago, Illinois published their study on the MIND Diet, a diet specifically formulated to benefit the brain by combining two diets—the Mediterranean diet, discussed on page 88, and the DASH diet, which was originally developed to reduce hypertension but has been shown to improve cognitive function, as well.

Between 2004 and 2013, 923 subjects between the ages of 58 and 98 were tracked and asked to fill out a "food frequency questionnaire." The questionnaires were then analyzed to see how closely the subjects' eating patterns followed the MIND diet, which emphasizes ten "brain-healthy food groups": leafy green vegetables, other vegetables, nuts, berries, beans, whole grains, fish, poultry, olive oil, and wine. The diet recommends three daily servings of whole grains; a salad and one other vegetable every day; a daily glass of wine; poultry and berries at least twice per week; fish at least once per week; beans every other day; and daily snacking on nuts. In addition, it severely limits the consumption of five designated unhealthy foods, which include red meats, butter and stick margarine, cheese, pastries and sweets, and fried and fast foods.

Dr. Morris and her colleagues found that participants who rigorously adhered to the MIND diet lowered their risk of AD by as much as 53 percent. Those who followed the diet only moderately still benefited with a 35-percent lower risk. The researchers emphasized that the results need to be confirmed by studies of different populations, as well as through randomized trials.

CALORIE-RESTRICTIVE DIETS

The idea that a calorie-restrictive (CR) diet can have health benefits first emerged in the 1930s, when researchers at Cornell University determined that low-calorie diets could extend the lives of rats. Later, in the 1990s, researchers discovered that calorie restriction can also have lifespan-extending effects on other animals—roundworms and fruit flies. Studies on monkeys have yielded similar results. The scientists who analyzed the results believed that by stressing the body, these diets activate biological programs in the cells that protect the animals against disease and degeneration. Meanwhile, as discussed in Chapter 2 (see page 57), the Okinawa Centenarian Study revealed that caloric restriction is in part responsible for the longevity and healthy aging enjoyed by the residents of Okinawa, Japan—so calorie restriction appears to benefit humans as well as animals.

In a 2009 issue of *PNAS* (Proceedings of the National Academy of Sciences of the United States of America), A.V. Witte and colleagues published the findings of the first human study showing that calorie restriction improves memory in the elderly. Fifty healthy normal or overweight subjects between the ages of 50 and 80 were divided into three groups. The first group was instructed to achieve a 30-percent reduction in caloric intake over a period of three months. To avoid malnutrition, a minimal intake of 1,200 calories a day was set. The second group was instructed to achieve a 20-percent increase in unsaturated fatty acids, which have been shown to boost brain health in animal studies. Members of the third group—the control group— were instructed to not change their previous eating habits. Both before and after the three-month study, all of the subjects were tested for memory performance.

After three months, researchers found a significant improvement in memory performance in the group that had adhered to a calorie-restricted diet, with benefits being most pronounced in the individuals who had best adhered to the CR diet. In the other two test groups, there were no significant changes in memory performance. The cognitive improvement in the calorie-restricted group was associated with decreased insulin levels; increased insulin sensitivity and, thus, reduced insulin resistance; and reduced inflammatory activity. These physiological changes were believed to stimulate neuroprotective pathways in the brain, thus preserving brain cell function over time. The researchers emphasized a need for further studies that would examine the impact of dietary changes on cognitive health.

THE FINGER STUDY

Because health is known to be affected by factors other than diet, one study was designed to investigate whether multiple interventions could improve cognitive function. Called the Finnish Geriatric Intervention Study to Prevent Cognitive Impairment and Disability, or the FINGER study, it was conducted over a two-year period, and the results were published in 2015 in *The Lancet* by Miia Kivipelto of the Karolinska Institutet in Stockholm, Sweden.

In this landmark study, 1,260 people between the ages of 60 and 77—all of whom were deemed to be at risk of dementia—were randomly assigned to two groups. The experimental group received high-intensity interventions, which included customized diet plans, strength training and aerobic workouts, computer-based cognitive training, management of vascular risk factors, and increased social interaction. The customized diets included high amounts of fruits and vegetables; cereals made with whole grains; low-fat dairy products and meat; vegetable oils (no butter); and fish at least twice per week, with a moderate intake of alcohol. The control group received only regular advice on the importance of healthy eating, physical activity, mental stimulation, and social activity. Mental function was measured both before and after the study period.

The Many Benefits of Overnight Fasting

On page 96, you will learn that the Alzheimer's Prevention and Treatment Diet includes several nights a week of fasting—in part, as a means of limiting the consumption of carbohydrates. While this may strike you as a radical idea, in recent years, intermittent fasting has been widely studied and found to have a beneficial effect on a broad array of body functions and systems.

Intermittent fasting—sometimes called *time-restricted eating*—describes the practice of restricting your eating to a small window of time each day. A 2013 review of studies designed to examine this dietary pattern, published in the *British Journal of Diabetes and Vascular Disease*, presented evidence that intermittent fasting may:

- Limit inflammation.
- Improve metabolic efficiency and reduce weight in obese individuals.
- Reduce LDL ("bad") cholesterol and total cholesterol levels.
- Help prevent, slow, and reverse type 2 diabetes.
- Improve pancreatic function.
- Improve insulin levels and insulin sensitivity.
- Reproduce some of the cardiovascular benefits associated with exercise.
- Protect against cardiovascular disease.
- Reduce blood pressure.
- Modify levels of harmful visceral fat.

After two years, researchers found that the experimental group's overall cognitive scores were 25 percent higher than those of the control group. The difference between the two groups was even more pronounced when the researchers focused attention on certain specific functions. The experimental group's executive function (the ability to get things done) was 83 percent higher than that of the control group, and its processing ability (the speed at which motor and brain functions can be performed together) was 150 percent higher. Findings also suggest that people with the APOE4 gene may actually benefit more from these interventions, showing again that we can indeed

The benefits just listed reveal several reasons why the eating pattern recommended in the APT Diet helps protect the brain. As you learned in Chapter 2, obesity, insulin resistance, type 2 diabetes, and cardiovascular disease are all associated with Alzheimer's disease. By helping avoid, reduce, or even reverse these conditions, restricted eating—even when the diet followed isn't ideal—can enhance brain health. When the diet is improved to include brain-protective foods like omega-3-rich fish and low-glycemic fruits and vegetables, the benefits can be even greater.

Why does restricted eating improve body function in so many ways? Some experts have suggested that our modern dietary habits place us in a continuous "feast mode." Because we eat meals and snacks nearly from the time we wake up until the moment we go to bed, the body is almost continually using glucose. As a result, it has adapted to burning sugar as its primary fuel. Intermittent fasting may "reboot" the metabolism so that the body can burn fat as its primary fuel. This not only promotes weight loss but also improves insulin sensitivity, which, as you know, is one of the keys to brain health.

Different patterns of intermittent fasting have been suggested by different studies. At the Alzheimer's Prevention Clinic, we have found that fasting overnight five nights a week is feasible for most people and can be easily integrated into their lifestyle over time. They can skip the nighttime fasts on weekends—they can even make occasional dietary slips—and still enjoy greater overall health and added brain support.

take control of our brain health in effort to win the "tug of war" against our genes. Follow-up studies will examine whether the group's boosted mental acuity will lower the risk of Alzheimer's disease and dementia.

THE APT DIET

The Alzheimer's Prevention and Treatment (APT) Diet takes into consideration all of the latest evidence on AD—including the studies cited in this chapter—and is also augmented in a variety of ways.

The APT Diet is best characterized as including omega-3-rich fish at least twice per week; skinless light-meat poultry at least four times a week, with no restrictions on the number of weekly servings; lean beef or pork no more than once a week; four to eight eggs per week; one or two servings of low- or no-fat dairy each day; one to three servings of whole grains each day; several servings of dark leafy greens, cruciferous vegetables, and other low-glycemic vegetables each day; and at least one serving per day of low- to moderate-glycemic fruit, including several servings of berries each week. Perhaps most important, we advise our patients to slowly reduce their daily consumption of carbohydrates to 100 to 120 grams per day. This is done in part by slowly increasing the nighttime period during which food is not eaten, so that eventually, carbs are avoided five nights a week for twelve to sixteen hours.

We have already discussed the reason for the restriction of carbohydrates. This strategy has been found to improve diet in a number of brain-healthy ways—by providing overall caloric restriction, by stimulating mild ketosis, and by improving glucose metabolism and insulin sensitivity. The foods featured in the diet, from dark leafy greens to omega-3-rich fish, have also been chosen because of their brain-healthy attributes. Other aspects of the diet have been geared to maximize your ability to stick to the food plan. After all, what good is a brain-healthy diet if people don't follow it? Because many individuals have a hard time cutting down their carb intake, the process of restricting carbs is gradual and is partly accomplished overnight, maximizing the chance of achieving success. (To learn about additional benefits of fasting overnight, see the inset on pages 94 to 95.) Fruit is strategically suggested as an after-meal dessert or a between-meals snack, providing a naturally sweet replacement for sugary desserts. This allows you to promote better brain health without sacrificing enjoyment.

After years of experience in working with patients, we know that no matter how motivated you are, you need practical assistance and encouragement when following a diet. That's why we created the Alzheimer's Universe website (www.alzU.org) to help educate and support Alzheimer's patients and their families, and the AD-NTS, or Nutritional Tracking System (www.alzheimersdiet.com/alzu), which allows patients to track their progress over time.

CONCLUSION

In this chapter, we have given an overview of some of the most important diets that have been studied as a means of preventing or treating Alzheimer's disease. We have also provided a brief discussion of the Alzheimer's Prevention and Treatment Diet, which we have used to improve the cognitive health of many hundreds of people who are at risk for AD or are already experiencing the effects of this disorder.

In the next chapter, you will learn more about the APT Diet as we review its guidelines; look at the best foods to include, as well as those that should be avoided; and learn how to maintain a brain-healthy eating plan.

5.

The APT Diet

In previous chapters, you learned how certain foods can support brain health. Now it's time to put that information into action. In the pages that follow, we outline a nine-week diet plan that will help get your brain health on track. But the benefits of the diet plan don't end after the nine weeks are up. It's important to understand that the habits you form during this period are meant to be maintained indefinitely. By eating right, fasting, exercising regularly, and adopting an overall brain-healthy lifestyle, you can make a real and lasting impact on your memory and cognitive function.

Believe in yourself! As we said in Chapter 4, this program is designed to be easy to follow, maximizing your ability to succeed. It starts off slowly, encouraging you to do something small but meaningful to improve your diet every day. What's more, it is a largely forgiving system that teaches you to cultivate healthy behaviors over the long term. Once you get used to practicing these behaviors on a regular basis, they will become second nature—you won't even think about them! What is vital is that you commit to taking the first step toward improving your brain health by making incremental changes over time.

If you are thinking about taking on this nine-week program, it is essential that you consult with your personal physician. The APT Diet is, on the whole, very much in line with dietary suggestions for common conditions like cardiovascular disease, diabetes, and high cholesterol. However, it is important to keep your treating physician aware of any plans to change your diet. Your doctor will be able to take your medical history into account, identifying any issues that might make it unwise or impractical for you to follow our recommendations. For example, certain diabetics who are predisposed to *ketoacidosis*—a serious condition that involves high blood sugar and high ketone levels—should not attempt to undertake a diet with periodic extended fasting. Again, we stress: For best results, and to avoid any negative health consequences, the nine-week diet plan should be followed *only* under the supervision of your treating physician.

For those people who have already been diagnosed with mild cognitive impairment (MCI) due to AD or dementia due to AD, modifications of the nine-week diet may be necessary. Weight management and the maintenance of muscle mass are key considerations

Calorie Considerations

The APT Diet does not suggest a set target for daily caloric intake. Instead, it focuses on making balanced dietary choices that support brain health according to current evidence. The most commonly used dietary guidelines state that women should generally aim for about 2,000 calories a day, and men should aim for 2,500 calories. On the APT Diet, calories tend to be lower, making them in line with studies which show that calorie restriction has positive effects on the brain.

It's important to note, however, that the APT Diet detailed in this chapter—and exemplified in the Sample Menus that start on page 153—is targeted for a person of average body weight, average percentage of body fat, average muscle mass, and moderate activity level. Individuals who have low to average body weight, a low percentage of body fat, average to high muscle mass, and higher activity levels can increase their food intake. Those with high body weight, high percentage of body fat, average to low muscle mass, and low activity levels may need to decrease their food intake and increase their exercise.

How can you learn your percentage of body fat or muscle mass? In the Alzheimer's Prevention Clinic, we use sophisticated equipment to

once the symptoms of AD appear. For example, if the person with AD is of normal or low body weight, it is essential that he or she avoid losing weight, which may occur in the course of the nine-week diet. It is especially important to avoid losing muscle mass. That's why we suggest seeking regular medical evaluations with a treating physician and, if necessary, consulting with a nutritionist. (See Chapter 7 for more information on adjusting the Alzheimer's Prevention and Treatment Diet for individuals with AD.)

CUSTOMIZING YOUR DIET AND MONITORING YOUR PROGRESS

Although we urge you to follow the week-by-week recommendations presented in this chapter, we understand that in some cases, a health condition may make it unwise to follow them to the letter. If you are

---

measure these factors. An alternative is to use at-home tools like body fat scales or to make use of a gym, personal trainer, or physician who has the necessary equipment and can track your progress over time. As discussed on page 53 of Chapter 2, the most harmful type of fat is visceral fat, which is stored around the internal organs. One measurement that approximates the amount of visceral body fat using only a tape measure is the waist-to-hip ratio. While there are several methods of calculating this ratio, one commonly used option is to first measure the narrowest part of your waist (midway between your hip and your rib cage) and then measure the largest area around the hips. Then, simply divide the circumference of your waist (in inches or centimeters) by the circumference of your hips. The target ratio for men is less than .9, and the target ratio for women is less than .85.

If any of your measurements—your weight, percentage of body fat, waist-to-hip ratio, etc.—indicate a potential problem, appropriate dietary modifications and exercise should help you reach a healthier number. We highly recommend that in such a situation, you work with a qualified healthcare professional and/or a registered dietitian who can provide guidance and oversee your progress. (See the discussion above for more information about customizing your diet.)

experiencing a health issue, work with your doctor so that the two of you can modify our recommendations as needed.

For some people, the changes recommended by the diet may have to be made over a longer period of time. For example, in Week 2, we ask you to limit your carbohydrates to 140 to 160 grams a day. But if you have been consuming 200 to 300 grams of carbs a day up until now, it may be too challenging to meet your carb target on Week 2. In that case, we suggest decreasing your carb intake over a period of several weeks until you meet your Week 2 goals. If, on the other hand, your present carbohydrate intake is *less* than that prescribed for Week 2, we do not suggest increasing it to the 140-to-160-gram range. Customize your diet as needed with the goal of eventually adhering to the guidelines provided for Week 9 as closely as possible.

Finally, if you find it too difficult to follow the program, we suggest that—rather than taking an all-or-nothing approach—you modify the diet as needed. Perhaps you can't reduce your carbohydrates to the level we've recommended, or maybe you can't incorporate three brain-healthy meals into your daily routine. Simply reduce your carbs as much as you comfortably can, and try to eat one or two brain-protective meals each day. With time and practice, you will start making better food choices more often.

As you follow the APT Diet, we encourage you to monitor your progress, using either the Nutrition and Activity Logs that begin on page 237 of this book or the Alzheimer's Disease-Nutrition Tracking System (AD-NTS) found on the Alzheimer's Universe website (www.AlzheimersDiet.com/alzu). There, you can record the most vital elements of the APT dietary approach by tracking carbohydrate intake, exercise, and brain-healthy snack and meal consumption. By consistently keeping an eye on your dietary and lifestyle habits, you'll be more attuned to how you eat and act from day to day. This will make it easier to stay on track.

AN OVERVIEW OF THE ALZHEIMER'S PREVENTION AND TREATMENT DIET

Over the course of the nine-week plan, you will gradually be implementing a number of basic changes to your lifestyle, setting the stage for a lifelong commitment to healthy habits. Of these habits, there are two that are the most important. One is that you will be reducing your total carbohydrate intake over time to between 100 and 120 grams a day. The second is that, several times a week, you will be undertaking an overnight fast with the ultimate goal of fasting five nights a week for a minimum of twelve and as many as sixteen hours. Throughout the nine-week diet—and afterwards—you should also be choosing your foods carefully, opting for the freshest and healthiest. (See "Your Final Dietary Goals," below.) When you do buy packaged foods, pay close attention to the Nutrition Facts labels of the products you choose, scanning for any brain-unhealthy components such as high carbohydrate counts, trans fats, and added sugars. (See the inset on reading a food label on page 104.)

By the time you've finished the nine-week diet, you will have hopefully adjusted your diet to the point where you're sticking to the following guidelines. Note that on page 112, after the list of dietary goals, you'll find a list of lifestyle goals that have been shown to protect brain function and can interact with good nutrition to maximize beneficial effects. While these goals may now seem intimidating, keep in mind that during your nine-week diet, you will work toward achieving them *gradually*.

Your Final Dietary Goals

Later in this chapter, you will learn the details of what you can eat each week of the nine-week Alzheimer's Prevention and Treatment Diet. (See page 115.) At this point, it's helpful to have an overview of your final (i.e., Week 9) dietary goals so that you will know what you're aiming for on the APT Diet. (For lists of recommended proteins, grains, vegetables, fruits, and more, see the inset on page 124.)

■ **Maximize your consumption of high-quality protein, each day eating at least 1 gram of protein for every 2 pounds of body weight.** Follow these guidelines when choosing proteins:

● **Eat skinless white meat chicken or turkey at least four times a week, with no upper limit as long as you stay within your calorie limits.** Skinless dark meat chicken is also acceptable in moderation,

Reading a Nutrition Facts Label

You'll have the greatest success following the Alzheimer's Prevention and Treatment Diet if your meals feature mostly fresh foods—lean poultry, meats, and fish cooked in as little brain-healthy fat as possible; fresh vegetables; fresh fruits; and whole grains (used in moderation). But, of course, in this busy world, we all rely on some packaged foods. As mentioned in this chapter, whenever choosing foods, you'll want to read the Nutrition Facts label and the ingredients list to make sure that the product is in keeping with your dietary goals. If you're not used to reading this label, it can be a little confusing—but it doesn't have to be. By understanding the Nutrition Facts label and using it in conjunction with the list of ingredients, you'll be able to choose products that work well with your diet and help support brain health. The following will guide you through the different components of the label.

Serving Size. Be sure to compare the manufacturer's serving size with what you are actually eating. If the manufacturer's serving size is 1 cup but you're eating 2 cups, you'll be getting twice as many calories, carbs, etc. as those stated on the Nutrition Facts label.

Calories (per serving). If you are trying to lose or gain weight, your healthcare provider may have you use a daily calorie budget. Once you know your budget, by keeping the manufacturer's serving size in mind, you'll be able to see how the product fits in your diet.

Fat Calories. This number tells you how many of the calories in the product are contributed by fat. Your diet should get no more than 35 percent of its calories from fat each day.

Percentage Daily Value. For some dietary components, such as total fat and cholesterol, the amount is expressed not only in grams or milligrams, but also as a percentage of the Daily Value figures, a recommended amount based on a diet of 2,000 calories. When reading these figures, keep in mind that if your calorie budget is more or less than 2,000 calories, these percentages will not hold true for you.

Total Fat. As you learned in Chapter 3 (see page 82), good fats are a valuable tool in the fight against Alzheimer's disease. Nevertheless, fat

Nutrition Facts

Serving Size: 1 cup (120 g)

Servings Per Container: 6

Amount Per Serving

Calories 150   **Fat Calories** 20

% Daily Value*

Total Fat 2g	3%
Saturated Fat 0g	0%
Trans Fat 0g	
Polyunsat Fat 0.5g	
Monounsat Fat 0.5g	
Cholesterol 0mg	0%
Sodium 210mg	9%
Potassium 160mg	5%
Total Carbs 32g	11%
Dietary Fiber 3g	11%
Soluble Fiber 1g	
Sugars 9g	
Protein 4g	

Vitamin A	15%
Vitamin C	0%
Calcium	10%
Iron	20%
Thiamin	20%
Riboflavin	20%
Niacin	20%
Vitamin B$_6$	20%
Folic Acid	20%
Phosphorus	10%
Magnesium	8%

*Percent Daily Values are based on a 2,000 calorie diet. Your daily values may be higher or lower depending on your calorie needs.

		Calories	2,000	2,500
Total Fat	Less than		65g	80g
Sat Fat	Less than		20g	25g
Cholesterol	Less than		300mg	300mg
Sodium	Less than		2,400mg	2,400mg
Potassium			3,500mg	3,500mg
Total Carbs			300g	375g
Dietary Fiber 25g			30g	

Figure 5.1. The Nutrition Facts Food Label.

is richer in calories than carbohydrates and protein, so you'll want to limit your fat consumption. Just as important, do your best to avoid trans fats, instead choosing products made with poly- and monounsaturated fats. (See below.)

Saturated Fat. Most experts feel that it is important to be mindful of saturated fat intake. On the Alzheimer's Prevention and Treatment Diet, we suggest that you limit your saturated fat consumption to about 10 percent of your total dietary intake. Note that your target may depend on a variety of medical and genetic factors, so talk to your doctor for a more precise recommendation.

Trans Fats. Since trans fats are considered the most harmful dietary fats (see page 80), you will want to eliminate *all* trans fats from your diet, so look for 0 grams trans fats. Because the manufacturer can claim zero trans fats as long as there's less than half a gram present, you should also check the listed ingredients to ensure that the product doesn't include any hydrogenated or partially hydrogenated oils, the most common sources of trans fats in commercial products.

Polyunsaturated Fat and Monounsaturated Fat. Both polyunsaturated and monounsaturated fats are considered heart-healthy, and are, for the most part, brain-healthy, as well. Look for products whose fats are derived from these two categories rather than the saturated fat category. Because some polyunsaturated fats, like corn oil, should not be eaten in excess, double-check the ingredients to ensure that the fats come from brain-healthy sources. (For more information on fats, see page 79.)

Cholesterol. According to the most recent USDA Dietary Guidelines, cholesterol is no longer a nutrient of concern for overconsumption. In the past, the recommended daily limit for cholesterol—which is found only in animal products—was 300 milligrams per day. However, the latest scientific research has not found a relationship between dietary cholesterol intake and actual cholesterol levels in the blood.

Sodium. The recommended daily limit for sodium is 2,300 milligrams per day. Ask your doctor if you need to further limit sodium because of a condition such as high blood pressure—which is associated with a higher risk of Alzheimer's disease. Keep in mind that many processed foods have high sodium counts, so it pays to check the values listed on the Nutrition Facts label.

Potassium. The recommended amount of potassium for a healthy adult is 4,700 milligrams per day. In the case of some conditions, such as kidney disease, potassium has to be kept at a lower level.

Total Carbs. The Alzheimer's Prevention and Treatment Diet limits carbohydrates, so every day, you'll want to keep your eye on your carbohydrate count. In the second week of the diet, you'll be aiming for no more than 140 to 160 grams of carbohydrates per day. By Week 9, you'll be limiting yourself to 100 to 120 grams of carbohydrates a day.

Dietary Fiber. Because fiber slows the digestion of food, and therefore helps prevent spikes in blood glucose levels, it makes sense to choose high-fiber foods whenever possible. You should get most of your fiber from leafy greens and other low-glycemic vegetables, berries and other low-glycemic fruits, and whole grains. When choosing packaged foods, try to select products that provide a good amount of fiber, aiming for 25 to 35 grams of fiber per day from food. As they age, many people require fiber supplementation to maintain regularity. Check with your doctor for a more personalized recommendation.

Sugars. Sugars causes blood glucose spikes that can lead to glucose intolerance, which has been associated with a higher risk of Alzheimer's disease. Limit sugar-laden foods like cookies, and restrict your daily intake of added sugars, ideally to less than 50 grams a day of your total grams of carbs.

Protein. Remember that the APT Diet recommends a rich amount of protein each day. (See the full discussion on page 76.) If you're not a vegetarian, most of this protein should come from skinless white-meat poultry, lean red meat, fish, and eggs. If you're a vegetarian, you'll be able to get your protein from soy products, legumes, grains, and vegetables.

Nutrients. The Nutrition Facts label provides information on the vitamin A, vitamin C, calcium, and iron contents of a food, although—like the label shown in Figure 5.1—it may also list information on other nutrients, such as iron, phosphorus, and magnesium. In the case of this food label, the product supplies substantial amounts of thiamin (B_1), riboflavin (B_2), niacin (B_3), and vitamin B_6, all of which are important for brain health. These values are expressed as a percentage of Daily Values, the recommended daily amount based on a 2,000-calorie diet. As the label states, your needs may be higher or lower for certain nutrients.

Ingredients. This part of the label, which is not found in the Nutrition Facts section, lists the product's ingredients in order of quantity. The ingredients listed first are present in the highest amount. So if sugar, high-fructose corn syrup, or white flour is the number-one ingredient, you'll know that this isn't the best product for the APT Diet.

although many experts believe that white meat chicken, with its lower fat content, provides more "bang for the buck" nutritionally.

● **Eat fish rich in omega-3 fatty acids at least twice a week.** Good choices include salmon, mackerel, lake trout, herring, sardines, and albacore tuna. Do not fry fish, and do not eat large amounts of shellfish, which is not technically within the "brain healthy" category—although, in moderation, it can serve as a reasonable source of protein. The recommended serving size is 6 ounces.

● **Eat lean grass-fed beef or lean pork no more than once a week.** The recommended serving size is 6 ounces.

● **Eat four to eight eggs per week.** Research has not told us exactly how many eggs we can eat each week and still maintain good health, but it *has* told us about the rich supply of nutrients contained in every egg. For most people, four to eight eggs a week are not only safe, but also beneficial. Depending on your protein and nutritional needs as well as your health status, you may be able to eat more than eight each week. (Discuss this with your doctor.) Keep in mind that although egg yolks contain saturated fat and cholesterol, studies have *not* shown that egg yolks raise cholesterol or increase the risk of heart disease. When possible, choose eggs from free-range chickens.

● **Eat low- and nonfat dairy in moderation, preferably from grass-fed cows.** Aim for one or two servings or so per day—preferably 6 ounces of low-fat Greek yogurt, with live and active cultures, plus 4 to 8 ounces of 1-percent milk or 1 to 2 ounces of low-fat cheese. Try to minimize non-grass-fed regular or full-fat dairy products to no more than six servings a week. We emphasize dairy products made with milk from grass-fed cows because research shows that these products are higher in healthy omega-3 fatty acids. (See page 171 to learn about omega-3 fatty acids.)

● **If you are a vegetarian, eat plentiful portions of the brain-healthy proteins discussed in Chapter 3 (see page 78).** Good choices include nuts and legumes (chickpeas, black-eyed peas, lentils, lima beans, kidney beans, pinto beans, soy beans, and black beans). A serving size of legumes is $1/2$ cup cooked. A serving of nuts is about one ounce, but check the label for the serving size. Because legumes are an easy way to optimize protein and fiber intake, nonvegetarians, too, should have several servings of legumes a week. Quinoa is another great high-protein option.

■ **Eat heart-healthy fats, and avoid or minimize fats that can damage your heart and blood vessels.** Follow these guidelines:

● **Eat moderate amounts of monounsaturated fats.** Choose olive oil as your primary oil, and aim for about 1 tablespoon a day, with a maximum daily intake of about 2 tablespoons a day. Also have a few servings of nuts a week (about one ounce or a small handful each), such as hazelnuts and almonds, and enjoy half an avocado a few times a week. These foods are rich in heart- and brain-healthy fats.

● **Be mindful of your consumption of saturated fats.** Aim for a *maximum* of 10 percent of your total daily calories. To achieve this, eat only lean meats; choose skinless white-meat poultry; limit butter and other full-fat, non-grass-fed dairy products; and limit fried foods and fast foods to no more than one meal a week—preferably, zero times a week).

● **Limit butter, cream, and mayonnaise to less than one 1-table-spoon serving a day.**

● **Avoid all trans fats.** To steer clear of this heart-damaging fat—which is found in packaged foods, especially baked items—do not buy any products that contain partially hydrogenated fats or oils.

■ **Eat only 100 to 120 grams of carbohydrates a day, emphasizing low-glycemic choices on as many days a week as possible—ideally, five or more.** Follow these guidelines when selecting carbs:

● **Eat moderate amounts of whole grains: one to three servings per day of whole grains and whole-grain breads and cereals that are high in fiber and have a relatively low glycemic index.** A serving size is 1/2 cup of grains or cereals or 1 slice of bread.

● **Eat at least one serving a day of leafy green vegetables (the more, the better); and at least one serving a day of cruciferous vegetables, such as broccoli and cauliflower, or other vegetables** that are low-glycemic, such as bell peppers, mushrooms, onions, green beans, and zucchini. A serving size is 1 cup raw or $\frac{1}{2}$ cup cooked.

● **Eat at least one serving of whole low- or moderate-glycemic fruit each day.** Two to four servings a week of berries, especially strawberries and blueberries, is strongly suggested. A serving size is $\frac{1}{2}$ cup. Avoid juicing and other methods of preparation that remove the healthy fiber, and be cautious of "smoothies," which can be made with tons of added sugar.

● **Limit added sugars to less than 50 grams a day.** When it comes to sugar, less is more! Eating refined sugar increases cravings for carbohydrates, especially higher-glycemic carbs. Some experts feel strongly that the lower-carb approach of the APT Diet is more easily followed when sugar intake is minimized. Whenever possible, rather than using table sugar, sweeten your food with agave syrup, which is a low-glycemic product that does not cause blood sugar to spike.

● **Limit pastries, sweets, and ice cream to no more than two times a week, and make portions as small as possible.**

■ **Limit fast foods and fried foods to no more than one meal a week.**

■ **Include caffeinated coffee, tea, and purified dark cocoa powder regularly.** One to three cups of caffeinated coffee (about 12 ounces a day) has been shown to have brain-protective effects. Decaffeinated coffee is perfectly fine, but there is more evidence in support of caffeinated coffee. If you prefer, drinking tea also appears to be beneficial, but there is more evidence in support of coffee. For its antioxidant effects, add dark cocoa powder to your coffee, yogurt, or low-sugar smoothie. Your goal is to add 375 to 650 milligrams of cocoa flavanols per day. Check the package, or consider using CocoaVia, which has been studied in clinical trials. Start with a small amount to insure that you can tolerate it, and slowly increase it over the weeks. (Some people experience side effects such as mild headaches.) Since pure dark cocoa is bitter, you will probably have to add a little sweetener to your coffee—preferably agave syrup, which is low-glycemic.(For more information about cocoa flavanols and cocoa powder, see page 173.) Just make sure to stay within your added-sugar limit of under 50 grams a day. To avoid interfering with sleep, try to avoid caffeinated beverages after lunchtime.

- **Drink alcohol in moderation.** Women should stick to one serving a day; men, to two servings. Most experts suggest a 5-ounce serving of red wine for optimum brain health, but it is unclear which type of alcohol is best. Other serving options include a 12-ounce beer (but watch the carbohydrate content!) or a 1.5-ounce shot of hard liquor.

- **Maximize your intake of antioxidants.** Keep your diet high in dark leafy greens, berries, coffee, tea, and dark cocoa powder, which are rich in brain-healthy antioxidants. See the previous recommendations regarding these foods.

- **Use fresh foods whenever possible, and when you do buy packaged foods, make smart ingredient choices.** You have already learned about some of the ingredients you should avoid, like trans fats, refined flour, and sugar. You'll also want to select foods with as few ingredients as possible—the fewer, the better. Finally, stick to ingredients you recognize. If you can't pronounce an ingredient or you don't know what it is, choose a different product.

- **At least three nights a week, avoid eating for twelve to fourteen hours—between dinner and breakfast—if tolerated. For two nights a week, avoid eating for fourteen to sixteen hours, if tolerated.** Note that water, tea, and other nonalcoholic, noncaloric beverages are fine during your fast. Avoid artificial sweeteners. (See the inset on page 112.) While most people can tolerate this period of caloric deprivation, be sure to discuss it with your doctor before attempting it. If you have any symptoms of dizziness, weakness, or lightheadedness, stop fasting. Also, if you have a medical condition such as diabetes and are prone to diabetic ketoacidosis, caution must be taken, and approval by your treating physician is necessary.

Artificial Sweeteners and the APT Diet

Over the last several years, more and more evidence has shown that artificial sweeteners may not be ideal when it comes to your health. While this is a complicated topic with some uncertainty, the APT Diet does not support the routine use of these sweeteners. A variety of studies have shown that a higher intake of these substances is associated with an increased risk of metabolic syndrome, weight gain, type 2 diabetes, and stroke.

You will do a service to both your overall health and your brain health if you satisfy your sweet tooth with naturally sweet whole fruit, with an emphasis on low-glycemic choices. (See the inset on page 125.) If you need to add a sweetener to beverages like coffee and tea, try to use only a small amount of a lower-glycemic sweetener like agave syrup, and limit added sugars to less than 50 grams a day.

Your Lifestyle Goals

Research has shown that in addition to a brain-healthy diet, a combination of beneficial habits—including exercise, staying mentally active, and alleviating stress—can reduce your risk of Alzheimer's. Work on incorporating the following habits slowly into your life, and your brain will reap the benefits.

Engage in Regular Physical Activity

Unless you are already following a sound exercise program, it's essential to increase your physical activity as tolerated and as approved by your primary care physician. Exercise increases blood flow to the brain and body, and reduces and helps manage the risk factors for cognitive decline, such as high cholesterol, high blood pressure, and diabetes. We recommend that you exercise at least three to four times a week for 45 to 60 minutes per session. Although research hasn't conclusively shown the optimal amount and type of exercise for brain protection, a mix of cardiovascular exercise (also known as cardio or aerobic exercise) and resistance/weight training is suggested for a target of between 160 minutes and 180 minutes a week. We also recommend that, if possible, you measure your body fat percentage, waist size, and weight every month or so. (See the inset on page 100 for more about these measurements.) If you are already physically active, it is essential to maintain your muscle mass over time. If you have been less active, you probably need to regain your muscle mass. As we age, it is common for body fat percentage to rise and lean muscle mass to fall. Fighting that decline is essential for optimal brain health. If motivation is a problem, consider hiring a personal trainer who will work with you each week. Dedicated time for exercise is essential and *required* if you are going to enhance your brain health. Finally, when sitting for extended periods of time, consider using a balance ball or a "stand-up" desk like an Ergotron standing work station to keep more muscles in use throughout the day. (See page 178 in Chapter 6 for a more in-depth discussion of exercise.)

Practice Good Sleep Hygiene

Studies have shown that sleep cleanses the brain of beta-amyloid, a substance that is known to accumulate in the brains of patients with Alzheimer's disease. For that reason, we strongly suggest sleeping at least seven and a half to eight hours every night. To optimize your ability to fall asleep, avoid texting, checking email, or using any electronics that emit a blue light for thirty to forty-five minutes before going to bed. A blue artificial light has been shown to prevent the release of melatonin, a hormone that reduces alertness and helps induce sleep. Also try to go to bed and wake up at the same times every day, avoid over-the-counter sleep aids such as Tylenol PM, and, as mentioned earlier, avoid drinking caffeinated beverages after lunchtime. While prescription sleep medications are widely used, emerging evidence suggests a possible relationship between some of these medications and the development of AD. More research is needed to clarify this point. Additionally, if you suffer from sleep apnea—which is characterized by excessive daytime sleepiness and snoring at night—it is strongly recommended that you see a qualified medical professional, like a sleep specialist. When sleep apnea is present, treatment is suggested to minimize the negative effects of nightly oxygen deprivation to the brain. (To learn about the use of medication to treat insomnia, see page 207 in Chapter 7.)

Keep the Brain Engaged

Learning something new is one of the best ways to keep your brain functioning. Try learning a new language (or brushing up on a language you used to speak); studying a new subject; or taking up a new hobby, especially in a group setting. Choose an activity that you truly enjoy, and stick with it. Also try to increase socialization, either on a one-to-one basis or through local activity programs, adult education classes, or clubs. Research shows that people who engage in frequent social interaction tend to maintain their brain vitality. These interactions are especially effective when they combine physical, mental, and social activities. (To learn more about increasing mental activity and socialization, see page 183 of Chapter 6.)

Learn to Play a Musical Instrument

Creating music requires complex neural activities that help build back-up pathways in the brain, which are essential for delaying cognitive decline and preserving brain health. It's therefore not surprising that this pastime has been associated with a reduced risk of Alzheimer's disease. Continue to play a musical instrument, learn to play one for the first time, or pick up an instrument that you used to play—and play regularly. If possible, take regular music lessons or join a local musical group, as this will make healthful social activities part of the experience. When choosing any activity, musical or otherwise, focus on those you enjoy rather than those you find frustrating or unpleasant.

De-Stress!

Stress can take a heavy toll on the brain, hampering the growth of nerve cells, causing shrinkage of the hippocampus (the memory portion of the brain), increasing your risk of Alzheimer's disease, and speeding the progression of AD. People with hectic work lives should note that every four to five years of work stress lead to one *additional* year of brain aging. Clearly, minimizing stress throughout your life is essential to protecting your brain function. Choose a stress-reducing method—whether yoga, meditation, acupuncture, or mindfulness training—and integrate it into your life. To more fully reduce stress, take periodic vacations, at least every three to four months, even if it's just a long weekend. (To learn more about stress and AD, see page 187 of Chapter 6.)

Participate in Ongoing Education

If you haven't done so already, sign up for a free account at the Alzheimer's Universe website (www.AlzU.org). This site was created by Weill Cornell Medicine and New York-Presbyterian and collaborators from throughout the world, and provides a variety of lessons and activities available to help you optimize and understand a comprehensive approach to brain-health. You will begin by completing a five- to ten-minute questionnaire, followed by lessons and activities. The more lessons you complete, the more will "unlock," and the more you will learn about overall brain health.

THE NINE-WEEK DIET PLAN

Now that you're familiar with the basic dietary and lifestyle principles of the Alzheimer's Prevention and Treatment Diet, you're ready to embark on the nine-week plan. Yes, this program will require a little effort and time. But as you will soon see, it's fairly easy to implement because it allows you to make healthy changes *gradually*. During Week 1, in fact, you will make no dietary or lifestyle changes at all. Instead, you will consider your dietary habits and begin learning more about the foods you usually eat so that you can start making better-informed choices. You will also plan ways in which you can make your daily activities more supportive of cognitive health—as well as more satisfying. Then, over the succeeding weeks, you will introduce modifications, making a few more changes each week.

While we have designed our program to have the highest rate of success possible, we recognize that you may not be ready to fully commit to every aspect of it right away. That's okay, because doing even a little bit to improve your brain health is better than doing nothing at all. Most important is that you commit to improving your brain health and begin taking action, bit by bit. Our nine-week diet plan is meant to start you on the road to success.

WEEK 1 OF THE APT DIET

During Week 1, you will not make any changes to your usual diet and lifestyle. Rather, you will take stock of your current situation—what foods you have in your house and what foods you generally eat—and figure out what you have to do to start making your life more brain-healthy. The availability of foods in your home has an enormous effect on what you eat. Fill your kitchen with junk foods, and you'll find it nearly impossible to avoid eating sugar- and fat-laden snacks. Fill your kitchen with fresh fruits and vegetables, lean proteins, whole grains, and other smart choices, and you're bound to improve your diet just because you've made good food readily available.

During this transition period, become more accustomed to reading Nutrition Facts labels and ingredient lists on packaged foods in preparation for Week 2. (See the inset on page 104.) In other words, this week is mostly about constructing the foundation of a brain-healthy life. The weeks that follow will build on this foundation.

Some people are eager to begin making healthy dietary changes right away. If you are ready to "jump in," don't feel that you have to wait! Finish the preparatory work described below, and immediately start the "Diet for Week 2," as detailed on page 122. Follow the Week 2 dietary guidelines for two weeks before moving on to Week 3.

Planning and Preparation for Week 1

- Identify three favorite brain-unhealthy snacks and three favorite brain-unhealthy meals that you eat on a fairly regular basis. Running late to work and need to grab a snack on the go? A jelly donut and an iced double four-pump mocha dulce latte cappuccino with heavy cream do not qualify as brain-healthy! No time for lunch? Two slices of pizza and a fountain soda provide more carbs and saturated fat than your body needs. These are just a few of the many potential snacks and meals that, when eaten regularly, are not compatible with optimal brain health. Record this information on the Nutrition and Activity Logs that begin on page 237 or on the Alzheimer's Diet-Nutrition Tracking System (AD-NTS). This will provide a record of the largest dietary "offenders," which you will replace with brain-healthier alternatives in the coming weeks.

- Look through your pantry and refrigerator, and identify all the foods that don't support healthy eating, such as sugar-laden snacks, refined-carbohydrate processed foods, and fatty foods like potato chips. Come up with some solutions. For instance, you will toss out all the foods that don't support the APT Diet, and you will not buy them again or will purchase them only occasionally and in limited quantities. (Consider donating unopened nonperishable foods to your local food bank.) Record this information on your log sheets or on the AD-NTS.

- Inform your family and close friends about the changes you will be making to accommodate your new brain-healthy diet. This serves three purposes. First, household members will expect changes in the home food environment and know why they're being made. Second, the process of changing your diet will be easier and more fun when the people around you are supportive. Third, once you announce these changes, you will feel accountable to others and will be more likely to stick with your plan. Overhauling your diet takes a whole team approach, and having those closest to you on your side will give you a greater chance for dietary success.

- When you go food shopping, pick up three brain-healthy snacks. (See the inset on page 118 for ideas.) Remember that you're going for low-carb, high-protein, nutrient-rich foods, so check the Nutrition Facts labels for grams of sugar, protein, etc.

Diet for Week 1

- Do not make any dietary changes yet. Just become more aware of your current habits and think about how you're going to replace the foods in your kitchen with foods that will support a brain-healthy diet.

- Read the Nutrition Facts labels and ingredients list on *every* food item you buy or eat. This will make you more familiar with your

Brain-Healthy Snacks

Brain-healthy snacks will help you feel satisfied throughout the day while nourishing and protecting your brain. You'll find a variety of wholesome snacks below, and many—like yogurt, nuts, and hummus—will boost your daily protein intake while providing other important nutrients. Remember that snacks count as part of your diet, so always choose your between-meal treats with your daily carbohydrate limit in mind.

- 1 slice whole-grain bread topped with 1 tablespoon peanut butter or other nut butter, such as almond or cashew. (Look for brands with no added sugar.)

- $\frac{1}{2}$ cup fresh strawberries, blueberries, raspberries, or blackberries.

- $\frac{1}{2}$ cup or one whole medium fruit other than berries, including apples, apricots, grapefruit, oranges, peaches, and plums. (For a more complete list of brain-healthy fruit, see the inset on page 125.)

- $\frac{1}{4}$ cup almonds, walnuts, or hazelnuts.

- 1 stick low-fat string cheese.

- 1 container (6 ounces) low- or nonfat yogurt, Greek or regular, preferably from grass-fed cows.

- 5 whole-grain crackers, such as Wheat Thins or Triscuits, topped with 1 ounce reduced fat cheese, if desired.

- Unlimited raw veggies (carrots, cucumber, broccoli, celery, grape tomatoes, or cauliflower) with $\frac{1}{4}$ cup yogurt-based dip, hummus, or guacamole.

- $\frac{1}{2}$ cup low-fat cottage cheese (preferably grass-fed).

- Unlimited celery sticks with 2 tablespoons nut butter.

- $\frac{1}{2}$ avocado drizzled with fresh lemon juice or hot sauce.

- $\frac{1}{2}$ cup cooked quinoa.

- 1 or 2 hard-boiled eggs (preferably from free-range chickens).

- 1 cup steamed or boiled edamame (young soybeans), lightly sprinkled with salt.

- 3 deli-thin slices (about 2 ounces total) roast turkey or chicken, spread with spicy mustard and rolled up. (If desired, roll in some shredded lettuce or other veggies for more fiber and nutrients.)

current diet so that you understand what you'll have to do to make better food choices. (See the inset on page 104 to learn how to read a Nutrition Facts label.)

● Most people eat far more carbohydrates than they realize. Since a major key to protecting your brain health is reducing your carb intake, it's vital that you become aware of the amount of carbs you're eating now. For two days—one weekday and one weekend day—write down everything you eat, and note the carb count for each item. If you're eating packaged foods, it will be easy to find the carbohydrate grams per portion listed under Nutrition Facts. If you're eating fresh food or food that for some other reason isn't accompanied by nutrient counts, look up the counts on the USDA's Supertracker website. (See page 232 of the Resources list.) Finally, total your carbs for each day, and record the totals on the Nutrition and Activity Logs on page 239 or on the AD-Nutrition Tracking System found on the Alzheimer's Universe website. We think you'll be amazed by the amount you're eating—way more than the 100 to 120 grams that is your Week 9 goal.

Lifestyle and Exercise for Week 1

● Check and record your weight to set your baseline, using a scale that you will have access to over the coming weeks. Ideally, you should check your weight every few weeks—at Weeks 4 and 7, for instance—always at the same time of day (preferably morning). Now is also a great time to determine your body fat percentage, if the necessary tool is available to you. If not, you can at least measure your waist and hip circumference and approximate your visceral fat. (See the inset on page 101 for directions.)

● Knowledge is power in the fight against AD. So, as first suggested on page 115, sign up for and complete the free online course at Alzheimer's Universe. Lessons are on a variety of topics, with a heavy emphasis on nutrition and lifestyle. They average five to ten minutes each, so they won't take up a lot of your time.

● With the help of your physician, a fitness instructor, or a personal trainer, identify and write down a number of exercises that could be safely performed for at least 20 minutes each, three times each week. As you consider potential exercises, keep three important things in mind:

First, if you are not very active at this point, when starting an exercise program, your activity should not be overly strenuous or require sweat or a gym to be effective.

Second, the benefits of exercise are cumulative, so although we ideally suggest setting aside a block of time for exercise, 5 minutes of increased activity performed four times a day is the same as 20 minutes performed at one time. (This could be as simple as committing yourself to taking the stairs instead of the elevator, walking briskly around the block one extra time, or getting in the habit of doing ten pushups before every shower.) If you are pressed for time, this strategy, combined with additional dedicated time built into your day, will give you the greatest chance for success.

Third, be sure to choose an activity that you find enjoyable. The more enjoyable the exercise, the more likely it is to be sustained long term. (See page 178 for more about exercise.)

The type and duration of your exercise may be recorded on the Nutrition and Activity Logs Found on page 237 or on the AD-NTS. This may also be a great time to consider a fitness tracking app or device. Many of these are free or already included on your cell phone, and they offer a good way of setting goals and monitoring progress over time. If you are already living an active lifestyle, keep it up! Maintain your program, try to increase it slowly over time, and diversify your experience so that your routine includes both cardio (aerobic) and resistance/weight exercises.

- Pick out a new activity that will keep your brain engaged, as discussed earlier in the chapter. (See page 114.) If you are not socially active, also think about ways in which you can become more involved with family, friends, or social groups within your community. If stress is weighing you down, think about ways in which you can release tension and create a mood of calm.

WEEK 2 OF THE APT DIET

During Week 2, you will start changing your home food environment, and you will try some new brain-healthy foods. You will also begin following the APT Diet, which—depending on how you've been eating—may require a big change in your shopping, food preparation, and eating habits, or may require only minor "tweaks."

Planning and Preparation for Week 2

- Revamp your home food environment. During Week 1, you identified the unhealthy foods that you had in your kitchen. Now it's time to make only foods that contribute to brain health readily available in your home. You should, of course, begin by throwing out potato chips, cookies, high-sugar cereals, and other foods that can damage your health. Then stock your kitchen with fresh fruits, vegetables, and other brain-protective foods. (For guidance, see the recommended foods inset on page 124.)

- Think about how you can retool any unhealthy meals you generally make so that they become brain-healthy. Instead of breading and frying dark-meat chicken, for instance, you can make or buy steamed, sautéed, or broiled skinless chicken breast. Instead of cooking up frozen French fries, steam some broccoli, spinach, or kale. Instead of drinking your favorite sugar-laden beverages as is from the carton or bottle, dilute them by mixing in some water and ice to reduce your daily carb intake. Experimenting with and finding several satisfying go-to brain-healthy meals is essential to making your brain and belly happy at the same time. (See the sample menus on page 153 for further ideas.)

- Purchase three new brain-healthy snacks, so that you now have a total of six brain-healthy snacks in the house. (See the inset on page 118 for snack ideas.)

- Purchase a variety of fresh low-glycemic fruits, especially berries, and low-glycemic vegetables. (See the lists on page 124.)

- Purchase at least one serving of omega-3-rich fish. (See the list on page 126.)

- Purchase dark cocoa powder. (See page 173.)

Diet for Week 2

This is the first week in which you'll be making changes in your diet, as detailed below. If you need lists of foods recommended on the APT Diet, turn to page 124; and if you need help putting together a day's worth of meals and snacks that follow Week 2's guidelines, refer to the sample daily menu on page 153. As you prepare and eat your meals, be sure to keep track of your carbohydrate intake by using either the Nutrition and Activity Logs that begin on page 237 or the AD-Nutrition Tracking System found on the Alzheimer's Universe website (see page 232).

- Limit carbohydrates to 140 to 160 grams per day.

- Eat at least 1 gram of protein for every 2 pounds of body weight (see page 76).

- Rely on light-meat skinless chicken, light-meat skinless turkey, and eggs as your primary source of animal-based protein. Use legumes, nuts, and seeds as your primary source of plant-based protein.

- Eat at least one serving of fatty fish (about 6 ounces each) this week.

- Eat no more than six servings (about 6 ounces each) of grass-fed lean red meat or pork this week.

- Eat at least one serving of vegetables ($1/2$ cup cooked or 1 cup raw each) each day.

- Eat at least two servings ($1/2$ cup each) of berries this week.

- Eat up to one additional serving ($1/2$ cup each) of other whole fruits per day.

- Eat two to four servings ($1/2$ cup each) of whole grains or whole wheat bread (1 slice each) per day.

- Eat one or two servings a day of low- or nonfat dairy, such as milk (8 ounces), cheese (1 or 2 ounces), and yogurt (6 ounces). Choose milk products from grass-fed cows when possible. Minimize the use of full-fat dairy products (no more than six servings this week).

- Use olive oil as your primary oil, and add further healthy mono-unsaturated fats to your diet by eating a few servings of nuts (one ounce each) and a few avocado halves during the week.

- Limit butter, cream, and mayonnaise to less than two 1-tablespoon servings a day.

- Limit fast foods and fried foods to no more than two or three meals this week.

- Limit pastries, sweets, and ice cream to no more than three or four servings this week, and make portions as small as possible.

- Have two or more servings a day of coffee, tea, or dark cocoa powder. (You can add the cocoa powder to your coffee. See page 173 for details.)

- Drink alcohol in moderation. Women should have no more than one serving a day; men, no more than two servings.

- Limit added sugars to less than 75 grams a day.

- As discussed in the inset on page 112, we do not advocate the consumption of artificially sweetened beverages. If you currently drink high amounts of these beverages, we suggest reducing your intake slowly over the next few weeks.

- At least two nights this week, avoid eating for at least ten to twelve hours between dinner and breakfast, if tolerated. Water, unsweetened tea, black coffee (decaffeinated), and other beverages without calories can be consumed during this period.

Lifestyle and Exercise for Week 2

- In the "Lifestyle and Exercise" portion of Week 1 (see page 119), you chose a few exercises that you could perform for 20 minutes each. This week, spend at least 20 minutes performing one of those exercises. If you generally exercise more than this, try to increase your activity by 20 minutes. Keep in mind that when you get to Week 9, your target will be 160 minutes of exercise, with a mix of cardio (aerobic) and resistance/weight training. After Week 9, we encourage you to increase your exercise to 180 minutes a week.

● In the "Lifestyle and Exercise" part of Week 1 (see page 120), you chose one activity that would help keep your brain engaged. This week, participate in that activity for at least one hour. If you have identified stress as a problem in your life, spend at least one additional hour using the stress-reduction technique of your choosing.

Recommended Foods for the Alzheimer's Prevention and Treatment Diet

The Alzheimer's Prevention and Treatment Diet emphasizes nutritious medium- to low-glycemic foods that have been shown to contribute to brain health. The following lists provide a handy guide to the best foods to include on your APT Diet.

RECOMMENDED VEGETABLES

Vegetables are an important part of any healthy diet. To feed and protect your brain, you'll want to stick to leafy green vegetables, cruciferous vegetables, and other low-glycemic vegetables. Choose from the lists below and follow the portion recommendations found on page 109.

Leafy Dark Green Vegetables

- Arugula
- Bok choy
- Chicory
- Collards
- Dandelion greens
- Kale
- Mustard greens
- Romaine lettuce
- Spinach
- Swiss chard
- Turnip greens
- Watercress

Cruciferous Vegetables

- Broccoli
- Brussels sprouts
- Cabbage
- Cauliflower
- Radishes of all types

Other Low-Glycemic Index Vegetables

- Artichoke hearts
- Artichokes
- Asparagus
- Bamboo shoots
- Bean sprouts
- Bell peppers
- Butternut squash
- Carrots
- Celery
- Cucumber
- Eggplant
- Garlic
- Green beans
- Leeks
- Mushrooms
- Okra
- Onions
- Pea pods
- Rutabaga
- Salad greens
- Sugar snap peas
- Summer squash
- Tomatoes
- Water chestnuts
- Zucchini

RECOMMENDED FRUIT

Fruit—especially berries—provide fiber and other important nutrients that have been shown to nourish and protect the brain. For optimum health, choose the low-glycemic berries and other fruits listed below, and follow the portion recommendations found on page 110.

Berries

- Blackberries
- Blueberries
- Boysenberries
- Raspberries
- Strawberries

Other Low-Glycemic Fruit

- Apples
- Apricots
- Cherries
- Grapefruit
- Guava
- Kiwi
- Mango
- Nectarines
- Oranges
- Peaches
- Pears
- Plums

RECOMMENDED GRAINS

Grains are high in fiber and other important nutrients, including the B vitamins and iron. To safeguard your brain, choose whole grains forms and, when possible, opt for one of the low-glycemic grains listed below. Always follow the portion recommendations found on page 109.

- Barley
- Brown rice
- Buckwheat
- Bulgur wheat (cracked wheat)
- Oats
- Quinoa
- Spelt
- Wild rice

RECOMMENDED PROTEINS

The Alzheimer's Prevention and Treatment Diet emphasizes protein, which is necessary for sound brain structure and function. Choose from among the following foods—which provide the protein you need without supplying a large amount of saturated fat—and follow the portion recommendations found on page 108.

- Skinless white-meat chicken, fat removed

- Skinless white meat turkey, fat removed

- Fish rich in omega-3 fatty acids, including salmon, mackerel, herring, lake trout, sardines, and albacore tuna

- Grass-fed lean beef, such as eye of round, top round, tip round, top sirloin, top loin, tenderloin, and 95-percent lean ground beef, fat removed when appropriate

- Lean pork, such as pork tenderloin, boneless top loin chops, pork top loin roast, pork center loin chop, pork sirloin roast, and pork rib chop

- Eggs (from free-range chicken, when possible)

- For vegetarians: Soy products, such as tofu and soy milk; legumes (see below); nuts (see below); and dairy products, if desired (see below)

RECOMMENDED DAIRY

Dairy products can be a good source of protein, calcium, and other nutrients, but they can also supply a large amount of saturated fat.

Select from the following low-fat and no-fat choices, and follow the portion recommendations presented on page 108. Ideally, choose products made with milk from grass-fed animals, and particularly avoid full-fat milk products unless they come from grass-fed sources. To support gut health, enjoy yogurt several times a week, or even daily, selecting yogurt with live and active cultures. (See page 63 of Chapter 2 to learn about the gut microbiome.)

- Nonfat or low-fat yogurt (regular or Greek, with live active cultures, but watch for added sugar!)
- Low-fat (1 percent) and fat-free (skim) milk from grass-fed sources
- Fat-free, reduced-fat, low-fat, and part skim hard cheeses
- Low-fat (1 percent) and nonfat soft cheeses, including low-fat and nonfat cottage cheese, farmer cheese, and part-skim or light ricotta

RECOMMENDED NUTS

All nuts are healthy because they supply heart-protective fats, protein, and vitamins and minerals, but the following nuts are especially nutritious. Just make sure to limit your portions (see page 108), as nuts are high in calories.

- Almonds
- Cashews
- Hazelnuts
- Macadamia nuts
- Pecans
- Pistachios
- Walnuts

RECOMMENDED LEGUMES

All legumes—which include beans, peas, and lentils—are good for you as they provide fiber, protein, iron, calcium, zinc, and B vitamins. The following are among the most nutritious legumes. Be sure to follow the portion recommendations found on page 108.

- Black beans
- Cannellini beans
- Garbanzo beans (chickpeas)
- Kidney beans
- Lentils
- Lima beans (butter beans)
- Navy beans
- Peanuts
- Peas
- Pinto beans
- Soybeans

WEEK 3 OF THE APT DIET

Now that your home food environment has been improved and some adjustments to your diet have been made, you should be ready for the more advanced dietary changes of Week 3. You will also continue the lifestyle modifications you began last week.

Planning and Preparation for Week 3

- Purchase ingredients for a new brain-healthy meal to replace a favorite brain-unhealthy meal. For some good ideas, refer to the Sample Menus on page 154.

- Pick one new exercise that could be performed for at least 20 minutes, three times each week. Your goal is to try different types of exercise until you find a few that you enjoy doing. You should also feel free to change off—doing different exercises on different days—to avoid boredom. If you have been thinking about joining a gym, now is a great time to take action. Also consider participating in group or team sports that may be available in your area.

Diet for Week 3

This week, you will continue making changes in your diet and will increase your nighttime fasts. Again, you can refer to page 124 if you need lists of suitable foods, and you can turn to page 154 for sample menus if you need guidance in creating snacks and meals that follow this week's guidelines. As you prepare and eat your meals, be sure to keep track of your carbohydrate intake by using either the Nutrition and Activity Logs that begin on page 237 or the AD-Nutrition Tracking System found on the Alzheimer's Universe website (see page 232).

- Limit carbohydrates to 140 to 160 grams per day.

- Eat at least 1 gram of protein for every 2 pounds of body weight (see page 76).

- Rely on light-meat skinless chicken, light-meat skinless turkey, and eggs as your primary source of animal-based protein. Use legumes, nuts, and seeds as your primary source of plant-based protein.

- Eat one to two servings of fatty fish (about 6 ounces each) this week.

- Eat no more than five servings (about 6 ounces each) of grass-fed lean red meat or pork this week.

- Eat at least one serving of green leafy vegetables ($\frac{1}{2}$ cup cooked or 1 cup raw each) each day, and at least one serving of cruciferous or other low-glycemic vegetables ($\frac{1}{2}$ cup cooked or 1 cup raw each) per day.

- Eat at least two servings ($\frac{1}{2}$ cup each) of berries this week.

- Eat up to one additional serving ($\frac{1}{2}$ cup each) of other whole fruits per day.

- Eat two to three servings ($\frac{1}{2}$ cup each) of whole grains or whole wheat bread (1 slice each) per day.

- Eat one or two servings a day of low- or nonfat dairy, such as milk (8 ounces), cheese (1 or 2 ounces), and yogurt (6 ounces). Choose milk products from grass-fed cows when possible. Minimize the use of full-fat dairy products (no more than six servings this week).

- Use olive oil as your primary oil, and add further healthy mono-unsaturated fats to your diet by eating a few servings of nuts (one ounce each) and a few avocado halves during the week.

- Limit butter, cream, and mayonnaise to less than two 1-tablespoon servings a day.

- Limit fast foods and fried foods to no more than two meals this week.

- Limit pastries, sweets, and ice cream to no more than three servings this week, and make portions as small as possible.

- Have two or more servings a day of coffee, tea, or dark cocoa powder. (You can add the cocoa powder to your coffee. See page 173 for details.)

- Drink alcohol in moderation. Women should have no more than one serving a day; men, no more than two servings.

- Limit added sugars to less than 70 grams a day.

- At least four nights this week, avoid eating for at least ten to twelve hours between dinner and breakfast, if tolerated. Water, unsweetened tea, black coffee (decaffeinated), and other beverages without calories can be consumed during this period.

Lifestyle and Exercise for Week 3

- Spend 20 minutes performing the exercise you used last week, and add an additional 20 minutes of your new exercise. If you are already more active than this, try to refine your regimen. Are you doing only or mostly cardio? Add one session of weight training at a minimum this week. Are you doing mostly weight or resistance training? Add one session of cardio at a minimum this week.

- Participate in last week's brain-engaging activity for at least one hour. If you have identified stress as a problem in your life, spend at least one additional hour using the stress-reduction technique of your choosing.

Maximize Exercise Success with a Fitness Buddy

You've already learned that physical activity is a vital part of a brain-healthy lifestyle. But perhaps, like many people, you find it difficult to stick to an exercise regimen. What's the solution?

Exercising with a fitness buddy is a great way to remain committed to physical fitness and have fun in the process. Fitness experts say that exercise partners provide a combination of motivation, support, and accountability. And, of course, they add brain-healthy socializing to your workouts. So consider asking a friend, neighbor, or family member to join you in your fitness sessions, or look for a reliable workout partner at your neighborhood gym. Studies show that this simple step can double your chance for fitness success.

WEEK 4 OF THE APT DIET

Week 4 builds on the dietary changes of the preceding week by further cutting carbs, adding more servings of certain brain-protective foods, and adding another night of fasting. You will also include an additional period of exercise in your week.

Planning and Preparation for Week 4

- Purchase ingredients for a new brain-healthy meal to replace a favorite brain-unhealthy meal.

- Plan for eating outside of the home. During the last two weeks, you probably ate at least some meals away from your home. Maybe it was easy for you, and maybe it was challenging. Now, give serious thought to healthy meals that you can prepare and pack for breakfast, lunch, and dinner when you're going to be away. After all, it's important to be able to enjoy nutritious brain-healthy foods wherever you go. Consider cooking more food for dinner the night before so that you have leftovers for the next day's meals, or buy wholesome prepared foods. Then consider the restaurants that you frequent, and think about healthy meals that you can order there for breakfast, lunch, and dinner. Remember that in most restaurants, you can have a favorite dish prepared a new way—fish can be sautéed instead of battered and fried, for instance, and instead of mashed potatoes, you can probably get cooked spinach, cooked green beans, or a salad. If you're given a large portion of meat or poultry—which is what most restaurants provide these days—have your server wrap half of it ahead of time so that you can take it home for tomorrow's lunch. Record this information so that you'll be able to stick to the APT Diet in just about any circumstances.

Diet for Week 4

This week, you will continue making changes in your diet and will increase your nighttime fasts. Again, you can turn to page 124 if you want to be sure of the foods recommended on this diet, and you can refer to the sample menus on page 155 if you need ideas for snacks and meals. Continue to keep track of your carbohydrate intake by using either the Nutrition and Activity Logs that begin on page 237 or the AD-Nutrition Tracking System found on the Alzheimer's Universe website (see page 232).

- Limit carbohydrates to 130 to 140 grams per day.

- Eat at least 1 gram of protein for every 2 pounds of body weight (see page 76).

- Rely on light-meat skinless chicken, light-meat skinless turkey, and eggs as your primary source of animal-based protein. Use legumes, nuts, and seeds as your primary source of plant-based protein.

- Eat at least two servings of fatty fish (about 6 ounces each) this week.

- Eat no more than five servings (about 6 ounces each) of grass-fed lean red meat or pork this week.

- Eat at least one serving, preferably several, of green leafy vegetables ($1/2$ cup cooked or 1 cup raw each) per day, and at least one serving of cruciferous or other low-glycemic vegetables ($1/2$ cup cooked or 1 cup raw each) per day.

- Eat two to three servings ($1/2$ cup each) of berries this week.

- Eat up to one additional serving ($1/2$ cup each) of other whole fruits per day.

- Eat two to three servings ($1/2$ cup each) of whole grains or whole wheat bread (1 slice each) per day.

- Eat one or two servings a day of low- or nonfat dairy, such as milk (8 ounces), cheese (1 or 2 ounces), and yogurt (6 ounces). Choose milk products from grass-fed cows when possible. Minimize the use of full-fat dairy products (no more than six servings this week).

- Use olive oil as your primary oil, and add further healthy monounsaturated fats to your diet by eating a few servings of nuts (one ounce each) and a few avocado halves during the week.

- Limit butter, cream, and mayonnaise to less than one 1-tablespoon serving a day.

- Limit fast foods and fried foods to no more than two meals this week.

- Limit pastries, sweets, and ice cream to no more than three servings this week, and make portions as small as possible.

- Have two or more servings a day of coffee, tea, or dark cocoa powder. (You can add the cocoa powder to your coffee. See page 173 for details.)

- Drink alcohol in moderation. Women should have no more than one serving a day; men, no more than two servings.

- Limit added sugars to less than 70 grams a day.

- On five or more nights this week, avoid eating for at least ten to twelve hours between dinner and breakfast, if tolerated. Water, unsweetened tea, black coffee (decaffeinated), and other beverages without calories can be consumed during this period.

Lifestyle and Exercise for Week 4

- Using the exercises you performed last week and adding a new one if necessary, increase your total amount of activity to 60 minutes this week, with roughly a two-to-one ratio of cardio to weight/resistance training—in other words, 40 minutes of cardio and 20 minutes of weight/resistance. Consider being evaluated by a physician and trying physical therapy if mobility issues prevent you from reaching your exercise goal. If you have joint limitations or arthritis, walking or swimming in a pool is a terrific low-impact exercise. If you are already more active than this, continue to refine your program. Think about hiring a personal trainer or taking exercise classes if you would like to learn more. If you haven't been integrating elements like yoga, Pilates, or spin classes, this would be a great time to give one of these activities a try.

- At the end of the week, check your weight again and, if the tools are available, check your percentage of body fat. (See the inset on page 101.)

- Participate in last week's brain-engaging activity for at least one hour. If you have identified stress as a problem in your life, spend at least one additional hour using the stress-reduction technique of your choosing.

Simple Ways to Reduce Stress During the Day

According to studies, stress can increase your risk of Alzheimer's disease. (See page 187.) But even during a busy day, there are simple things you can do to keep anxiety from taking a toll on your health. Here are a few essential practices:

- Breathe slowly and deeply. By oxygenating your blood, deep breathing can help you relax quickly. Just place your hand on your abdomen and inhale slowly through your nose so that your hand moves as your belly expands. Hold the breath for a few seconds, exhale slowly, and repeat.

- Visualize calm. Close your eyes, take several deep breaths, and imagine a relaxing scene, such as lying on a beach or walking through the woods. Focus on the details—the sights and sounds—and feel your stress melt away.

- Take a walk—even if it's just to your office water cooler. By forcing you to breathe more deeply, a walk can help soothe frayed nerves.

- Stroke your dog or cat. Even a few minutes of peaceful interaction with a pet has been shown to lower blood pressure and create a calmer frame of mind.

- Make plans for a special event, such as a weekend getaway or a movie. Looking forward to something provides perspective when things seem overwhelming.

WEEK 5 OF THE APT DIET

You are now halfway through the nine-week diet plan! Already, significant changes have been made to your home food environment, your daily diet, and your activity level. At this point, you should feel comfortable experimenting with new brain-healthy foods and guesstimating the carb content quickly and efficiently. One of the major changes this week involves increasing the duration of your overnight fast for twelve to fourteen hours, if tolerated. To help ease you into this change, the number of fasting nights per week has been decreased from five to four.

Planning and Preparation for Week 5

● Identify at least two challenges to brain-healthy eating outside the home. Then identify two potential solutions to each challenge, and record this information in your progress charts.

● Choose a new brain-stimulating activity that you would like to try, or try to enhance the activity that you have already begun. For example, if you recently picked up an instrument that you used to play and began experimenting with it, consider taking formal lessons with an instructor. If you began learning a new language through an audio-based course, consider planning a trip to a country that speaks the language as a way to reward yourself for your efforts and fine-tune your craft.

Diet for Week 5

This week, you will make minor changes in your diet and will increase the length of your nighttime fasts. Turn to page 124 if you need to view the list of recommended foods, and refer to the sample menus on page 156 if you want guidance in creating a day of snacks and meals that follow this week's guidelines. Continue to keep track of your carbohydrate intake by using either the Nutrition and Activity Logs that begin on page 237 or the AD-Nutrition Tracking System found on the Alzheimer's Universe website (see page 232).

- Limit carbohydrates to 130 to 140 grams per day.

- Eat at least 1 gram of protein for every 2 pounds of body weight (see page 76).

- Rely on light-meat skinless chicken, light-meat skinless turkey, and eggs as your primary source of animal-based protein. Use legumes, nuts, and seeds as your primary source of plant-based protein.

- Eat at least two servings of fatty fish (about 6 ounces each) this week.

- Eat no more than four servings (about 6 ounces each) of grass-fed lean red meat or pork this week.

- Eat at least one serving, preferably several, of green leafy vegetables ($^1/_2$ cup cooked or 1 cup raw each) each day, and at least one serving of cruciferous or other low-glycemic vegetables ($^1/_2$ cup cooked or 1 cup raw each) per day.

- Eat two to three servings ($^1/_2$ cup each) of berries this week.

- Eat up to one additional serving ($^1/_2$ cup each) of other whole fruits per day.

- Eat two to three servings ($^1/_2$ cup each) of whole grains or whole wheat bread (1 slice each) per day.

- Eat one or two servings a day of low- or nonfat dairy, such as milk (8 ounces), cheese (1 or 2 ounces), and yogurt (6 ounces). Choose milk products from grass-fed cows when possible. Minimize the use of full-fat dairy products (no more than six servings this week).

- Use olive oil as your primary oil, and add further healthy mono-unsaturated fats to your diet by eating a few servings of nuts (one ounce each) and a few avocado halves during the week.

- Limit butter, cream, and mayonnaise to less than one 1-tablespoon serving a day.

- Limit fast foods and fried foods to no more than two meals this week.

- Limit pastries, sweets, and ice cream to no more than two servings this week, and remember that the less sugary foods you eat, the better. Make portions as small as possible.

- Have two or more servings a day of coffee, tea, or dark cocoa powder. (You can add the cocoa powder to your coffee. See page 173 for details.)

- Drink alcohol in moderation. Women should have no more than one serving a day; men, no more than two servings.

- Limit added sugars to less than 65 grams a day.

- At least four nights a week, avoid eating any food for at least twelve to fourteen hours between dinner and breakfast, if tolerated. Water, unsweetened tea, black coffee (decaffeinated), and other beverages without calories can be consumed during each period of nighttime fasting.

Lifestyle and Exercise for Week 5

- If tolerated, perform the previously chosen exercises for at least four 20-minute periods for a total of 80 minutes per week. Remember to maintain a roughly two-to-one ratio of cardio to weight/resistance activities for maximum benefits. If you are already doing more exercise than this, keep it up!

- Participate in last week's brain-engaging activity for at least one hour, and consider either adding a new activity or enhancing your old one, as discussed on page 135.

- If stress continues to be a problem in your life, spend at least one additional hour each week using the stress-reduction technique of your choosing. If your stress has not been diminished by this technique or by the activity and lifestyle changes that you have been making over the last month, consider talking to your physician or to a counselor or therapist for added support. Be aware that some clinicians specialize in the treatment of stress and anxiety disorders.

WEEK 6 OF THE APT DIET

Week 6 will see further small dietary changes and will also increase your exercise sessions. Continue to add new brain-healthy meals and snacks to your diet. Also note any challenges that arise and find solutions to them as quickly as possible.

Planning and Preparation for Week 6

● Create and record one new brain-healthy meal so that you continue to add to your repertoire. This will make it easier and more pleasurable to follow the APT Diet.

Diet for Week 6

This week, you will make several minor changes in your diet, including a decrease in carbs, an increase in vegetables and berries, and less fast and fried foods. As always, you can turn to the sample menus on page 157 if you need guidance in creating a day of snacks and meals that follow this week's guidelines, and you can refer to page 124 for a list of recommended foods. Continue to keep track of your carbohydrate intake by using either the Nutrition and Activity Logs that begin on page 237 or the AD-Nutrition Tracking System found on the Alzheimer's Universe website (see page 232).

● Limit carbohydrates to 120 to 130 grams per day.

● Eat at least 1 gram of protein for every 2 pounds of body weight (see page 76).

● Rely on light-meat skinless chicken, light-meat skinless turkey, and eggs as your primary source of animal-based protein. Use legumes, nuts, and seeds as your primary source of plant-based protein.

● Eat at least two servings of fatty fish (about 6 ounces each) this week.

● Eat no more than four servings (about 6 ounces each) of grass-fed lean red meat or pork this week.

- Eat at least one serving, preferably several, of green leafy vegetables ($\frac{1}{2}$ cup cooked or 1 cup raw each) each day; and at least one serving, preferably several, of cruciferous or other low-glycemic vegetables ($\frac{1}{2}$ cup cooked or 1 cup raw each) per day.

- Eat two to four servings ($\frac{1}{2}$ cup each) of berries this week.

- Eat up to one additional serving ($\frac{1}{2}$ cup each) of other whole fruits per day.

- Eat one to three servings ($\frac{1}{2}$ cup each) of whole grains or whole wheat bread (1 slice each) per day.

- Eat one or two servings a day of low- or nonfat dairy, such as milk (8 ounces), cheese (1 or 2 ounces), and yogurt (6 ounces). Choose milk products from grass-fed cows when possible. Minimize the use of full-fat dairy products (no more than six servings this week).

- Use olive oil as your primary oil, and add further healthy monounsaturated fats to your diet by eating a few servings of nuts (one ounce each) and a few avocado halves during the week.

- Limit butter, cream, and mayonnaise to less than one 1-tablespoon serving a day.

- Limit fast foods and fried foods to no more than one meal this week.

- Limit pastries, sweets, and ice cream to no more than two servings this week, and make portions as small as possible.

- Have two or more servings a day of coffee, tea, or dark cocoa powder. (You can add the cocoa powder to your coffee. See page 173 for details.)

- Drink alcohol in moderation. Women should have no more than one serving a day; men, no more than two servings.

- Limit added sugars to less than 65 grams a day.

- At least four nights a week, avoid eating for twelve to fourteen hours between dinner and breakfast, if tolerated. Water, unsweetened tea, black coffee (decaffeinated), and other beverages without calories can be consumed during this period.

Lifestyle and Exercise for Week 6

- Perform at least 100 minutes of exercise this week. Continue the exercises that you have used in prior weeks, but try to increase each session's duration from 20 minutes to 30 minutes or more. Also add more variety and increase the weights used.

- Participate in last week's brain-engaging activity for at least one hour or, preferably, two hours. If stress remains a problem, continue using any stress-reducing techniques that seem to help. Also consider new techniques such as meditation or mindfulness training.

How Does Coffee Support Brain Health?

On page 110, we state that coffee has been found to have brain-protective effects. In fact, study after study has shown that regular coffee consumption reduces the risk of developing Alzheimer's disease.

How does coffee support the brain? Many researchers suspect that caffeine may play a major role. In addition to being a brain stimulant, caffeine blocks the receptors for a chemical called adenosine, which normally prevents the release of excitatory brain chemicals. When adenosine is blocked, brain-sparking chemicals flow more freely, potentially improving mental performance and slowing mental decline. Substances other than caffeine may also provide benefits. Coffee is a source of more than 1,000 different plant-derived chemical compounds, some of which have antioxidant and anti-inflammatory properties.

More in-depth research must be performed before we can understand the relationship between coffee use and AD prevention. In the meantime, studies support the use of moderate coffee consumption—one to three cups a day—as an effective weapon in the war against Alzheimer's disease.

WEEK 7 OF THE APT DIET

This week, you will continue much of last week's diet, but you will make further adjustments that move you toward brain-healthy meals. You will also again increase your weekly exercise time by 20 minutes for a total of at least two hours this week.

Diet for Week 7

During Week 7, you will maintain last week's carbohydrate limit, but will further limit added sugars and will increase your fasting. Turn to the recommended foods list on page 124 and to the sample menus on page 158 if you need guidance in creating a day of snacks and meals that follow this week's guidelines. And, of course, continue to keep track of your carbohydrate intake by using either the Nutrition and Activity Logs that begin on page 237 or the AD-Nutrition Tracking System found on the Alzheimer's Universe website (see page 232).

- Maintain last week's limit of 120 to 130 grams of carbs per day.

- Eat at least 1 gram of protein for every 2 pounds of body weight (see page 76).

- Rely on light-meat skinless chicken, light-meat skinless turkey, and eggs as your primary source of animal-based protein. Use legumes, nuts, and seeds as your primary source of plant-based protein.

- Eat at least two servings of fatty fish (about 6 ounces each) this week.

- Eat no more than three servings (about 6 ounces each) of grass-fed lean red meat or pork this week.

- Eat at least one serving, preferably several, of green leafy vegetables ($1/2$ cup cooked or 1 cup raw each) each day; and at least one serving, preferably several, of cruciferous or other low-glycemic vegetables ($1/2$ cup cooked or 1 cup raw each) per day.

- Eat two to four servings ($1/2$ cup each) of berries this week.

- Eat up to one additional serving ($1/2$ cup each) of other whole fruits per day.

- Eat one to three servings ($1/2$ cup each) of whole grains or whole wheat bread (1 slice each) per day.

- Eat one or two servings a day of low- or nonfat dairy, such as milk (8 ounces), cheese (1 or 2 ounces), and yogurt (6 ounces). Choose milk products from grass-fed cows when possible. Minimize the use of full-fat dairy products (no more than six servings this week).

- Use olive oil as your primary oil, and add further healthy monounsaturated fats to your diet by eating a few servings of nuts (one ounce each) and a few avocado halves during the week.

- Limit butter, cream, and mayonnaise to less than one 1-tablespoon serving a day.

- Limit fast foods and fried foods to no more than one meal this week.

- Limit pastries, sweets, and ice cream to no more than two servings this week, and make portions as small as possible.

- Have two or more servings a day of coffee, tea, or dark cocoa powder. (You can add the cocoa powder to your coffee. See page 173 for details.)

- Drink alcohol in moderation. Women should have no more than one serving a day; men, no more than two servings.

- Limit added sugars to less than 60 grams a day.

- At least five nights a week, avoid eating for twelve to fourteen hours between dinner and breakfast, if tolerated. Water, unsweetened tea, black coffee (decaffeinated), and other beverages without calories can be consumed during this period.

Lifestyle and Exercise for Week 7

- Add an additional 20 minutes of exercise to your regimen this week for a total of at least two hours. Congratulations! Two hours of weekly exercise is an accomplishment, and it will greatly contribute to both your brain health and your overall well-being. Continue the two-to-one ratio of cardio exercise to weight/resistance (about 80 minutes of cardiovascular and 40 minutes of weights).

- At the end of the week, check your weight again and, if the tools are available, check your percentage of body fat. (See the inset on page 101.)

- Continue participating in brain-engaging activities for at least one to two hours this week—and every week, going forward. Follow any stress-reduction techniques as needed.

Learning the Right Way to Weigh Yourself

On the Alzheimer's Prevention and Treatment Diet, we urge you to weigh yourself every few weeks to make sure that you are maintaining a healthy weight, and to use the same scale each time, as scales vary. The following tips will further help ensure that you get accurate results when you check your weight.

- Always weigh yourself at the same time of day—ideally, in the morning before breakfast. Weight can fluctuate as much as three pounds during the day.

- Don't weigh yourself after a big night out. Restaurant meals are usually large and full of salt, which makes you retain water. Wait at least a day before stepping on the scale again.

- Take fluids into account. Two eight-ounces glasses of water can add a pound of weight—temporarily, of course. After drinking a great deal of fluid, give yourself an hour or two before checking your weight.

- Don't weigh yourself directly after exercising. Exercise can cause fluid loss through sweat, which can make it seem that you've lost weight even when you haven't.

WEEK 8 OF THE APT DIET

This week, you will reduce your carbohydrate limit, increase your fasting, and continue your exercise sessions. By the end of this week, you will have nearly met your final dietary goals and will be ready for the last "tweaks" of your APT Diet.

Diet for Week 8

During Week 8, you will make minor dietary changes, including another decrease in your daily carb limit and an increase in your fasting time. Sample menus can be found on page 159 if you need help in creating a day of snacks and meals that follow this week's guidelines, and lists of recommended foods are found on page 124. Continue to keep track of your carbohydrate intake by using either the Nutrition and Activity Logs that begin on page 237 or the AD-Nutrition Tracking System found on the Alzheimer's Universe website (see page 232).

- Reduce your carbohydrate limit to 110 to 120 grams per day.

- Eat at least 1 gram of protein for every 2 pounds of body weight (see page 76).

- Rely on light-meat skinless chicken, light-meat skinless turkey, and eggs as your primary source of animal-based protein. Use legumes, nuts, and seeds as your primary source of plant-based protein.

- Eat two or more servings of fatty fish (about 6 ounces each) this week.

- Eat no more than two servings (about 6 ounces each) of grass-fed lean red meat or pork this week.

- Eat at least one serving, preferably several, of green leafy vegetables ($1/2$ cup cooked or 1 cup raw each) each day; and at least one serving, preferably several, of cruciferous or other low-glycemic vegetables ($1/2$ cup cooked or 1 cup raw each) per day.

- Eat two to four servings ($1/2$ cup each) of berries this week.

- Eat up to one additional serving ($1/2$ cup each) of other whole fruits per day.

- Eat one to three servings ($1/2$ cup each) of whole grains or whole wheat bread (1 slice each) per day.

- Eat one or two servings a day of low- or nonfat dairy, such as milk (8 ounces), cheese (1 or 2 ounces), and yogurt (6 ounces). Choose milk products from grass-fed cows when possible. Minimize the use of full-fat dairy products (no more than six servings this week).

How to Choose the Best Yogurt

Throughout this book, we encourage you to eat low- and no-fat yogurt, as this food provides protein and other important nutrients, as well as probiotics—healthy bacteria that are beneficial to the gut. But not all yogurts are created equal. To find the best yogurt for the APT Diet, follow these guidelines:

- Look for the Live and Active Cultures seal on the yogurt container. It lets you know that the product you're buying has at least 100 million cultures per gram.

- If you're struggling to meet your daily protein requirement, choose Greek yogurt, which has a higher protein content than regular yogurt.

- Be aware that some yogurts are loaded with sugar. Look for a product that has relatively little added sugar, or buy unsweetened yogurt and add a touch of honey or agave syrup. Skip products that have add-ins like granola and chocolate chips.

- Use the yogurt well within the expiration date, as the number of live bacteria tends to decline as the product sits on the shelf.

- Use olive oil as your primary oil, and add further healthy mono-unsaturated fats to your diet by eating a few servings of nuts (one ounce each) and a few avocado halves during the week.

- Limit butter, cream, and mayonnaise to less than one 1-tablespoon serving a day.

- Limit fast foods and fried foods to no more than one meal this week.

- Limit pastries, sweets, and ice cream to no more than two servings this week, and make portions as small as possible.

- Have two or more servings a day of coffee, tea, or dark cocoa powder. (You can add the cocoa powder to your coffee. See page 173 for details.)

- Drink alcohol in moderation. Women should have no more than one serving a day; men, no more than two servings.

- Limit added sugars to less than 55 grams a day.

- At least four nights this week, avoid eating for twelve to fourteen hours between dinner and breakfast, if tolerated. At least one night this week, avoid eating for at least fourteen to sixteen hours. Water, unsweetened tea, black coffee (decaffeinated), and other beverages without calories can be consumed during this period. While most people can tolerate this level of fasting, you should discuss this change with your doctor before implementing it. If you have any symptoms of dizziness, weakness, or lightheadedness, immediately stop the fast.

Lifestyle and Exercise for Week 8

- Perform your established mix of cardio and weight/resistance exercises for at least 140 minutes this week.

- Continue your brain-engaging activities and think about ways to get some of your friends and/or family involved in these activities, as well. Continue using stress-reduction techniques as needed.

WEEK 9 OF THE APT DIET

In the last week of the nine-week diet plan, you will be making one final reduction in your carbohydrate intake, increasing your exercise time to the weekly minimum, and making a final change in your fasting schedule.

Planning and Preparation for Week 9

- List your ten favorite brain-healthy snacks and meals eaten over the nine-week period. Turn to this list whenever you need snack and meal ideas so that you can continue following the APT Diet with greater ease.

Diet for Week 9

This week, you will make the final changes in your diet and reach your final dietary goals, as first outlined on pages 103 to 111 of this chapter. Sample menus can be found on page 160 if you need help in creating a day of snacks and meals that follow this week's guidelines, and lists of recommended foods can be found on page 124. For this last week, you should continue to keep track of your carbohydrate intake by using either the Nutrition and Activity Logs that begin on page 237 or the AD-Nutrition Tracking System found on the Alzheimer's Universe website (see page 232).

- Reduce your carbohydrate limit—for the last time—to 100 to 120 grams per day.

- Eat at least 1 gram of protein for every 2 pounds of body weight (see page 76).

- Rely on light-meat skinless chicken, light-meat skinless turkey, and eggs as your primary source of animal-based protein. Use legumes, nuts, and seeds as your primary source of plant-based protein.

- Eat two or more servings of fatty fish (about 6 ounces each) this week.

Using Meal Replacements

Ideally, we would all sit down to eat freshly prepared brain-healthy meals three times a day, every day. But in real life, busy schedules don't always allow us to do this. We urge you to think ahead and prepare simple meals—protein-packed, low-carb salads and sandwiches, for instance—that you can take with you to work and other activities, and to seek out restaurants and prepared-food stores where you can pick up nutritious meals when you're on the go. A little planning can go a long way toward helping you follow the APT Diet. But we also know that sometimes, you will be caught without a meal, and you may be tempted to resort to an unhealthy option like a fast-food burger or a slice of pizza. Fortunately, there is another alternative—meal replacements in the form of protein bars and protein shakes.

Protein bars can be purchased ready-made and kept in a pocket, desk drawer, or work bag, allowing you to grab one whenever you don't have access to a meal of freshly prepared foods. As you probably know, some nutrition bars are little better than glorified candy bars, containing tons of sugar, high fructose corn syrup, artificial colors and flavors, and other not-so-healthy ingredients. Be sure to look for bars with high-quality protein, heart-healthy fats, and wholesome, recognizable ingredients. If possible, minimize artificial sweeteners, too. Choose a bar that has a taste you enjoy and that provides nutrition which comes as close as possible to the guidelines provided below.

Optimal Nutrition in a Meal Replacement

Total Fat	5 to 10 grams for bars; 0 to 5 grams for shakes.
Saturated Fat	Less than half of total fat.
Carbohydrates	Less than 15 grams.
Sugar	Less than 5 grams.
Protein	1 gram of protein per every 10 calories.
Vitamins	Folic acid, B_6, B_{12}, and D.
Fiber	At least 5 grams.

When chosen carefully, protein bars provide sensible nutrition that will allow you to stick to the APT Diet and keep you satisfied until your next meal. Are these bars actually better for you than fast foods? The following comparison answers this important question. As you'll see, protein bars do a much better job of providing the protein you need without blowing your carb, sugar, and fat budgets.

Big Mac Burger versus Protein Bar

	Big Mac	Protein Bar
Calories	540	290
Total Fat (g)	28	9
Saturated Fat (g)	10	4
Carbohydrates (g)	47	14
Sugar (g)	9	4
Protein (g)	25	29
Fiber (g)	3	5

If you prefer shakes to bars, the most brain-healthy option is to make your own high-protein beverage. Simply place about eight ounces of low-fat milk or Greek yogurt in a blender, and process in a scoop or two of whey protein powder, a handful of berries or other low-glycemic fruit, and a handful or two of leafy greens or other low-glycemic veggies. (See the inset about protein powders on page 78.) Mix until well blended, and enjoy. This makes a wonderful on-the-go breakfast whenever you can spare a few minutes before leaving the house in the morning.

Remember that unprocessed whole foods—which have a brain-healthy balance of vitamins, minerals, and other micronutrients—are always your best bet for getting the nutrition you need. But when life gets hectic, a protein bar or shake can help you keep on track.

- Eat no more than one serving (about 6 ounces) of grass-fed lean red meat or pork this week.

- Eat at least one serving, preferably several, of green leafy vegetables ($1/2$ cup cooked or 1 cup raw each) each day; and at least one serving, preferably several, of cruciferous or other low-glycemic vegetables ($1/2$ cup cooked or 1 cup raw each) per day.

- Eat two to four servings ($1/2$ cup each) of berries this week.

- Eat up to one additional serving ($1/2$ cup each) of other whole fruits per day.

- Eat one to three servings ($1/2$ cup each) of whole grains or whole wheat bread (1 slice each) per day.

- Eat one or two servings a day of low- or nonfat dairy, such as milk (8 ounces), cheese (1 or 2 ounces), and yogurt (6 ounces). Choose milk products from grass-fed cows when possible. Minimize the use of full-fat dairy products to no more than six servings per week.

- Use olive oil as your primary oil, and add further healthy monounsaturated fats to your diet by eating a few servings of nuts (one ounce each) and a few avocado halves during the week.

- Limit butter, cream, and mayonnaise to less than one 1-tablespoon serving a day.

- Limit fast foods and fried foods to no more than one meal per week.

- Limit pastries, sweets, and ice cream to no more than two servings a week, and make portions as small as possible.

- Have two or more servings a day of coffee, tea, or dark cocoa powder. (You can add the cocoa powder to your coffee. See page 173 for details.)

- Drink alcohol in moderation. Women should have no more than one serving a day; men, no more than two servings.

- Limit added sugars to less than 50 grams a day.

- At least three nights a week, avoid eating for twelve to fourteen hours between dinner and breakfast, if tolerated. For two nights a week, avoid eating for fourteen to sixteen hours. Water, unsweetened tea, black coffee (decaffeinated), and any other beverages that have no calories can be consumed during this period. While most people are able to tolerate this level of fasting, you should discuss the fast with your doctor before attempting it. If you have any symptoms of dizziness, weakness, or lightheadedness, immediately stop the fast.

Lifestyle and Exercise for Week 9

- Increase your exercise to a minimum of 160 minutes a week, using the same two-to-one ratio of cardio to weight/resistance training.

- Participate in last week's brain-engaging activity for at least one hour. If you have identified stress as a problem in your life, spend at least one additional hour using the stress-reduction technique of your choosing.

SAMPLE MENUS FOR THE APT DIET

Throughout this chapter, you have learned about the overall principles of the Alzheimer's Prevention and Treatment Diet, as well as the specific guidelines for following the diet during Weeks 2 through 9. (No changes to the diet are made during Week 1.) The sample menus that begin on page 153 were designed to help you put the principles of each week into practice by suggesting one sample breakfast, lunch, and dinner, along with two healthy snacks.

Keep in mind that these menus were not intended to tell you what you *must* eat, but only to serve as examples of brain-healthy, satisfying meals and snacks that are consistent with the APT Diet. As long as you follow the basic principles we discuss in this book, you can choose whatever foods you wish from the recommended food lists that begin on page 124. At first, you may find it easier to follow the menus presented below but to swap out one recommended food for a food that you prefer. For instance, you might want to replace chicken with turkey or exchange a side dish of spinach and mushrooms for one of green beans. As you move through and beyond Week 9, we encourage you to personalize your menus as much as possible and to rework favorite recipes to make them more brain-healthy, as this will help ensure your long-term success.

At the end of the menus, you'll find a table that states the total calories, fat, carbohydrates, protein, dietary fiber, sugars, and added sugars for each day's meals. Based on your physician's recommendations, you may have to increase or decrease one or more of these macronutrients. For example, if you have been diagnosed with a kidney disorder, you may have to reduce the amount of protein you eat. The nutrient counts we provide will help you tailor your menus to meet your own dietary requirements.

The calorie count of each day's menu may seem low compared with current recommendations (see page 100), but as explained on page 92, it has been found that some calorie restriction may be beneficial for memory protection. If you need more calories, we suggest that you add another healthy low-carbohydrate snack to your day or that you increase portion sizes, especially of vegetables or of high-protein foods such as chicken, dairy, and nuts. This will help you get the calories you need while keeping your diet as brain-protective as possible.

You'll note that when we list coffee or tea, we don't mention common add-ins, like sugar or milk. Optionally, you may add one teaspoon of sugar—or, even better, some low-glycemic agave syrup—and/or one tablespoon of low-fat milk to your coffee or tea. The cocoa powder listed as part of each breakfast may be consumed at any time throughout the day, although due to its caffeine content, we suggest that you enjoy it in the morning so that it doesn't interfere with sleep. Because unsweetened cocoa powder is bitter, it's a good idea to stir it into coffee or yogurt. If it is still too bitter for your taste, try adding a little sweetener. (See page 173 to learn more about cocoa.)

When you read the sample menus, be aware that the portion sizes of meat, fish, and poultry refer to *cooked* portions of food. Because some weight is lost during the cooking process, we recommend that you start with an uncooked portion that is 1.5 to 2 ounces higher in weight. For instance, to end up with 6 ounces of baked chicken breast, you should start with approximately 7.5 ounces of raw chicken.

As we mention many times throughout this book, everyone's dietary needs are unique, so it is essential that you consult with your doctor and/or dietitian before beginning the APT Diet.

SAMPLE MENUS

WEEK 2

BREAKFAST

1/2 cup whole-grain cereal (such as bran flakes)

1/2 cup strawberries

4 ounces low-fat (1%) milk

4–6 ounces Greek or regular low-fat yogurt

1 cup coffee or tea

1 packet CocoaVia, or 1–2 teaspoons unprocessed,
unsweetened cocoa powder

MORNING SNACK

1 hard-boiled egg

1 medium apple

LUNCH

1 cup turkey chili with beans

1 ounce baked tortilla chips

1 fresh plum

AFTERNOON SNACK

8 celery sticks

2 tablespoons peanut butter

DINNER

6 ounces salmon, baked or grilled

3 small roasted red potatoes

1/2 cup green beans, sautéed in olive oil

WEEK 3

BREAKFAST

2 large eggs, scrambled or fried in olive oil

2 turkey sausage links or patties

1/2 grapefruit

8 ounces low-fat (1%) milk

1 cup coffee or tea

1 packet CocoaVia, or 1–2 teaspoons unprocessed,
unsweetened cocoa powder

MORNING SNACK

I slice whole wheat bread spread
with 1 tablespoon almond or other nut butter

LUNCH

Black beans and rice (1/2 cup cooked black beans,
1/2 cup cooked brown rice)

Sliced raw bell peppers (unlimited)
with 1/4 cup hummus

1/2 cup blueberries

AFTERNOON SNACK

1 ounce reduced-fat Cheddar cheese

5 whole-grain crackers (such as Wheatables,
Wheat Thins, or Triscuits)

DINNER

6 ounces lean pork, baked or grilled

2 cups kale or mixed greens, tossed with 2 tablespoons
olive oil vinaigrette

1/2 cup steamed or mashed cauliflower

WEEK 4

BREAKFAST

½ cup regular or steel-cut oats, cooked in water

½ cup mixed berries

4–6 ounces Greek or regular low-fat yogurt

1 cup coffee or tea

1 packet CocoaVia, or 1–2 teaspoons unprocessed,
unsweetened cocoa powder

MORNING SNACK

½ cup low-fat cottage cheese

1 small peach (or ½ cup canned juice-packed peaches)

LUNCH

Salade Nicoise (2 cups lettuce, 5 ounces water-packed
canned tuna, 1 sliced tomato, ½ cup green beans,
8 medium black olives, tossed with 2 tablespoons
balsamic vinegar and oil)

½ whole wheat bagel spread with 1 tablespoon
light cream cheese

AFTERNOON SNACK

¼ cup mixed nuts

DINNER

6 ounces skinless turkey breast, baked or grilled

½ cup steamed broccoli

½ medium baked sweet potato topped with 1 tablespoon
butter or trans-fat-free spread

WEEK 5

BREAKFAST

Berry Smoothie (1/2 cup Greek or regular low-fat yogurt, 1 cup fresh or frozen mixed berries, 1/4 cup orange juice)

1 cup coffee or tea

1 packet CocoaVia, or 1–2 teaspoons unprocessed, unsweetened cocoa powder

MORNING SNACK

1/4 cup almonds, raw or roasted

1 medium orange

LUNCH

1 cup butternut squash soup

5 whole-grain crackers (such as Wheatables, Wheat Thins, or Triscuits)

Raw veggies such as broccoli, snow peas, and celery (unlimited)

1/4 cup veggie dip made with yogurt

AFTERNOON SNACK

Meat and cheese roll-ups

(three 1-ounce slices deli turkey breast, 3 thin slices Swiss cheese)

DINNER

6 ounces lean beef, baked or grilled

1/2 cup each mushrooms and spinach, sautéed in olive oil

WEEK 6

BREAKFAST

1/2 cup whole-grain cereal (such as Kashi GoLEAN)

1/2 cup raspberries

8 ounces low-fat milk

1 cup coffee or tea

1 packet CocoaVia, or 1–2 teaspoons unprocessed,
unsweetened cocoa powder

MORNING SNACK

2 hard-boiled eggs

LUNCH

Turkey Wrap (whole wheat tortilla, 2 ounces deli turkey,
1/2 avocado sliced, 2 leaves romaine lettuce, 1 slice Swiss cheese,
2 teaspoons mustard, 1 tablespoon mayonnaise)

8 baby carrots

AFTERNOON SNACK

1/2 cup low-fat cottage cheese

1 medium tomato, sliced or chopped

DINNER

6 ounces chicken, baked or grilled

1 cup cooked spaghetti squash

1/2 cup homemade or no-sugar-added pasta sauce

1 cup raw kale tossed in balsamic vinegar and olive oil

WEEK 7

BREAKFAST

Berry Nutty Oatmeal ($\frac{1}{2}$ cup oatmeal cooked in water,
1 ounce chopped walnuts, $\frac{1}{2}$ cup blueberries)

4–6 ounces Greek or regular low-fat yogurt

1 cup coffee or tea

1 packet CocoaVia, or 1–2 teaspoons unprocessed,
unsweetened cocoa powder

MORNING SNACK

5 whole-grain crackers (such as Wheatables,
Wheat Thins, or Triscuits)

1 ounce harvarti or other white cheese

LUNCH

Tuna Salad (3 ounces water-packed canned tuna, 2 tablespoons
plain Greek yogurt, chopped onion, chopped celery)

$\frac{1}{2}$ whole wheat pita

2 pieces green leaf lettuce

Spinach Salad (1 cup raw spinach, 5 grape tomatoes,
1 tablespoon chopped bacon, if desired,
tossed in olive oil and vinegar)

5 fresh cherries

AFTERNOON SNACK

Raw radishes and celery (unlimited)

$\frac{1}{4}$ cup hummus

DINNER

6 ounces lean pork, baked or grilled

4 asparagus spears, steamed or sautéed in olive oil

$\frac{1}{2}$ cup cooked quinoa, seasoned with olive oil or butter

WEEK 8

BREAKFAST

2 eggs, boiled or poached

$1/2$ whole wheat English muffin,
spread with $1/2$ tablespoon butter or trans-fat-free spread

$1/2$ grapefruit

8 ounces low-fat milk

1 cup coffee or tea

1 packet CocoaVia, or 1–2 teaspoons unprocessed,
unsweetened cocoa powder

MORNING SNACK

$1/2$ cup blueberries

1 piece cheese (1 ounce or less),
such as Mini Babybel

LUNCH

Black and Blue Salad (3 ounces grilled lean steak strips,
2 cups red leaf lettuce, 2 tablespoons crumbled blue cheese,
$1/4$ cup slivered almonds, 2 tablespoons balsamic vinaigrette)

AFTERNOON SNACK

Raw sliced bell peppers and carrots (unlimited)

$1/4$ cup guacamole (mashed avocado and tomato)

DINNER

6 ounces salmon, baked or grilled

$1/2$ cup Brussels sprouts, roasted with olive oil

$1/2$ cup cooked brown rice

WEEK 9

BREAKFAST

Western Scramble (2 eggs scrambled, chopped peppers and onions,
2 ounces chopped ham, 1 ounce shredded mozzarella)

1 cup coffee or tea

1 packet CocoaVia, or 1–2 teaspoons unprocessed,
unsweetened cocoa powder

MORNING SNACK

4–6 ounces Greek or regular low-fat yogurt

1 peach

LUNCH

Greek Chicken Salad (3 ounces grilled chicken breast, 2 cups chopped
romaine lettuce, 1 ounce crumbled feta cheese, 1 tomato, chopped,
¼ cup sliced black olives, 2 tablespoons Greek vinaigrette)

AFTERNOON SNACK

½ avocado drizzled with lemon juice

¼ cup cashews, raw or roasted

DINNER

Mediterranean Pasta (1 cup cooked whole wheat pasta,
3 ounces cooked shrimp, 1 cup sautéed vegetables,
garlic, and olive oil)

2 cups kale or mixed greens,
tossed with 2 tablespoons lemon vinaigrette

Macronutrients for Each Week's Total Menus

Week Number	Total Calories	Total Fat	Total Carbs	Total Protein	Total Dietary Fiber	Total Sugars*	Added Sugars†
2	1,593	68 g	157 g	101 g	29 g	65 g	10 g
3	1,739	75 g	157 g	115 g	34 g	53 g	10 g
4	1,646	71 g	140 g	122 g	26 g	47 g	9 g
5	1,637	58 g	140 g	125 g	31 g	59 g	8 g
6	1,649	79 g	125 g	123 g	30 g	54 g	13 g
7	1,742	88 g	130 g	118 g	25 g	36 g	6 g
8	1,628	82 g	118 g	113 g	25 g	51 g	6 g
9	1,735	94 g	117 g	121 g	29 g	49 g	8 g

* "Total Sugars" are those sugars occurring naturally (such as in fruit or milk) plus those that are added to foods in processing.

† "Added Sugars" are only those added to foods in preparation and/or commercial processing.

BEYOND WEEK 9

Congratulations! You have made it through the nine-week diet program, dedicating significant effort toward changing your lifestyle. By this time, brain-healthy eating should be a matter of habit to you. You are now familiar with principles of the APT Diet and with the challenges associated with brain-healthy eating, both inside and outside the home. You should also have several strategies in place for dealing with those challenges. Your home should be stocked with a number of brain-healthy snacks and meal ingredients. Whenever you want to dine out, you should have a list of restaurants that can accommodate your needs, and you should know the most brain-healthy options available on each menu. Perhaps most important, you should be familiar with the nutritional content—especially the carbohydrates—of the majority of foods you eat.

After you have completed the nine-week diet plan, work on maintaining the program. Continue to limit your carbohydrate intake to 100 to 120 grams each day, and keep up your overnight periods of fasting five times a week. Eat at least two servings of fish each week; keep all of your proteins lean; and eat a bounty of fruits and vegetables, making low-glycemic choices whenever possible. If you can, increase your exercise time to an average of 180 minutes each week. That's only 180 minutes out of the 10,080 minutes you have each week!

As time goes on, you'll have to learn how to prepare for other possible obstacles to brain-healthy eating, such as vacations, holidays, and parties. You'll also want to prepare for stressful periods, such as moving and changing jobs. All of life's challenges can make it more difficult to follow any kind of diet. Think ahead, prepare early, and always carry a brain-healthy meal replacement for emergencies. (See page 148.) That way, nutritionally sound options will always be available to you.

Although it is important to remain aware of your diet, it is no longer necessary to formally document your meals and their carbohydrate content. If you encounter the dreaded diet fatigue—in other words, if you grow tired of the diet and revert to old habits—read this book again and focus on changing the practices that require the least noticeable sacrifice. Continue to experiment with new brain-healthy ingredients and meals. Do what you can to make this diet work for you. Remember that it's vital to keep your belly happy as well as your brain. You should love your food choices. Don't think about your eating patterns as a "diet" but rather as a new brain-healthy way of life!

6.

Other Strategies
for AD Prevention

D iet is one of the most important weapons we have in the fight against Alzheimer's disease. But in addition to changing the way you eat, there are a number of other steps you can take to support your brain health. We believe that a comprehensive *multi-modal* approach—that is, an approach that combines several different strategies and disciplines—is the best way to both prevent and treat Alzheimer's disease. Research shows that multimodal approaches create *synergy,* meaning that the benefits derived from the various strategies used in combination are greater than the sum of the separate benefits.

In one animal study, older beagles who undertook an antioxidant-rich diet, a twice-weekly exercise regimen, and an increased socialization program saw higher scores on cognitive tests than did dogs who received a standard diet and standard care. Perhaps more important, dogs who received the combination program were able to learn new tasks, outperforming not only dogs in the standard diet and care group, but also dogs who had received just the antioxidant diet or the exercise and socialization program. Clearly, having a wide-ranging and diverse approach to brain health is a good idea.

These results have been mirrored in human studies. The Finnish Geriatric Intervention Study to Prevent Cognitive Impairment and Disability (the FINGER study), first discussed in Chapter 4 (see page

93), offers some of the most compelling evidence to date that we can use a variety of techniques to take control of our brain health and see real advantages. The researchers found that older adults who participated in a program that provided customized diet plans, physical exercise, cognitive training, social activities, and cardiovascular health management performed significantly better on cognitive tests than did similar adults who received only general health advice.

Put simply, where Alzheimer's prevention and treatment is concerned, the whole is greater than the sum of the parts. In this chapter, we will discuss some of the best techniques you can use to round out your new brain-healthy lifestyle. By using carefully selected supplements; by becoming physically, intellectually, and socially active; and by reducing your level of stress, you can chip away at your risk of AD from all sides.

BRAIN-HEALTHY SUPPLEMENTS

As scientists delve deeper into new strategies for Alzheimer's prevention and treatment, much more attention has been given to supplements. Dietary supplements, also referred to as *nutraceuticals,* are vitamins, minerals, herbs, amino acids, and other substances that you consume in addition to your regular meals in order to maintain or encourage good health. They do not require a prescription from a physician—although some are also available by prescription—and can be purchased in supermarkets, health food stores, and drugstores, as well as online. Although research is still inconclusive in many cases, evidence indicates that certain supplements may be beneficial to brain health, helping to ward off or slow the progression of Alzheimer's disease and other dementias. In this section, we review the most promising of these supplements.

Be aware that it is not our intention to suggest that supplements can replace a healthy, balanced diet. Whole foods rich in brain-healthy vitamins, minerals, and other nutrients provide hundreds of naturally occurring substances that can help protect both your brain and your overall health. There is no miracle pill that will counteract the damaging effects of a diet high in sugar, trans fats, and saturated fats. In certain circumstances, though, supplements may be valuable to compensate for nutritional deficiencies or to provide additional benefits when used in conjunction with brain-healthy foods.

How do you know if a supplement is right for you? Before beginning any supplementation regimen, talk to your personal physician. Your doctor will be better able to determine whether you are deficient in any essential nutrients, and make recommendations based on your medical status and history. For example, if you are eating brain-healthy fish twice per week, and an otherwise balanced diet rich in omega-3 fatty acids, you may not need to take an omega-3 supplement. Your doctor can test your blood to see if your levels of omega-3 fatty acids DHA and EPA are optimal, or if there is room for improvement. Of course, minimum blood levels have not been established for all the supplements we're about to discuss, and it's worth pointing out that in some studies, people have derived cognitive benefits from supplements even when they were not experiencing deficiencies. That's why for each supplement, you should look at the possible benefits and weigh it against any risks. Then, in consultation with your physician, decide whether you want to add the supplement to your brain-healthy lifestyle.

New research is continually being published that increases our understanding of the effects of supplements on brain health. While an in-depth review of all of the potential vitamins and supplements that may (or may not) assist in protecting the brain is beyond the scope of this book, here we summarize the most practical, evidence-based, low-risk options. For reputable and up-to-date sources of information on this topic, visit the websites of the National Center for Complementary and Integrative Health and the Alzheimer's Drug Discovery Foundation. (See page 234 of the Resources list.)

Vitamins

In a perfect world, you would get all the vitamins you need through your diet alone. For a variety of reasons, this isn't always possible. Even when our hectic lifestyles allow us to eat brain-healthy meals on a regular basis, we sometimes fall short. Some individuals who are at risk for a vitamin deficiency due to a preexisting medical condition or a poor diet may have been advised by their doctor to take a specific

Buying Supplements

The quality of the vitamins and other supplements you buy will have a marked effect on the health of your body and, consequently, the health of your brain. To begin, it's important to know that there are four grades of supplements. From highest-quality to lowest, they are as follows:

Pharmaceutical grade. This grade meets the highest regulatory requirements for purity, dissolution (ability to dissolve), and absorption. Pharmaceutical grade supplements are 99-percent pure, with no binders, fillers, dyes, or other unknown substances. Quality is assured by an outside party—the United States Pharmacopeia (USP). This high quality does not come cheap, however. Pharmaceutical grade supplements can cost three times as much as supermarket supplements and are available only from compounding pharmacies, better health food stores, and doctors' offices. In some states, you need a prescription to obtain supplements of this quality.

Medical grade. These supplements are also high in quality, but may not meet all the standards for purity set by the USP.

Cosmetic or nutritional grade. Supplements of this grade are often not tested for purity, dissolution, or absorption, and may not contain the amount of active ingredients listed on the label.

Feed or agricultural grade. Supplements of this grade are produced for veterinary purposes and should not be used by humans.

To experience the full benefits of your nutritional supplement program, choose pharmaceutical grade products when available. A good health food store usually stocks supplements of several different grades. Ask which ones are pharmaceutical quality. Generally, medical trials are performed using pharmaceutical grade supplements, and dosage recommendations are based on these high-quality products. If you use a product of a lower grade, you may be getting far less of the active ingredient than you need for good results. For instance, a pharmaceutical grade omega-3 fatty acids supplement that states it contains "700 mg EPA" actually contains a full 700 mg EPA. If you buy a lower-quality product, a capsule marked "700 mg" may contain far less.

Throughout our discussion of supplements, we urge you to speak to your physician about the nutrients that you want to include in your brain-health program. Besides helping you choose the various nutrients, your doctor may be helpful in guiding you to the best brands. Several supplements may be available by prescription, which would help guarantee that the supplement provides exactly what is stated on the package label.

When buying supplements that are not of pharmaceutical grade, you still should look for the highest quality possible. The following guidelines should help you identify the purest and most effective products available:

- Look for supplements that contain no preservatives or artificial coloring—nothing but the nutrient itself. Be especially careful to avoid ingredients and fillers to which you have a sensitivity or allergy. Usually, the supplement label will let you know if that product contains soybeans, dairy, gluten, corn, and other ingredients that may be problematic.

- When possible, consider natural forms of nutrients rather than synthetic forms. Natural vitamin E, for instance, is better absorbed and more active than synthetic vitamin E.

- Be aware that many herbal supplements have been found to contain contaminants such as arsenic, lead, mercury, cadmium, and pesticides. Look for herbs that have a seal of approval from the United States Pharmacopeia (USP), NSF International, or ConsumerLab.com. These groups test products for label accuracy, lack of contamination, and the ability to dissolve and be absorbed by the body.

- Make sure that the supplement is packaged in a container that protects it from the light. Amber-colored glass is the best choice. When you purchase the nutrient, ask if it requires refrigeration.

- Choose products that have been vacuum sealed to preserve freshness. When you puncture the paper seal over the container, you should hear a mild popping sound indicating that the vacuum has been broken. Also make sure that the container has a tamper-proof seal.

vitamin, or a combination supplement like a multivitamin, to address that specific deficiency. The discussions below examine vitamins from the perspective of Alzheimer's prevention.

Multivitamins

Many people, including some doctors, believe that a multivitamin provides insurance against vitamin deficiency and poses no risks. But in the last few years, this assumption has been called into question. For most otherwise healthy people who maintain a balanced diet, recent evidence has shown that taking a multivitamin may not lead to additional health benefits. It can even be harmful.

Some research suggests caution when it comes to the supplemental intake of two minerals, copper and iron. In one study, people with the highest levels of copper were found to lose cognition three times faster than adults whose copper levels were normal. Iron is suspected of causing brain damage, as well—possibly because both copper and iron cause oxidative stress that injures neurons. Another study showed that when 1,450 people took cognition tests, those who performed highest had the lowest blood levels of copper and iron.

Copper and iron are both necessary for good health, as these nutrients work together to form red blood cells. But, as you've learned, too much of these metals may be harmful. Speak to your doctor about your copper and iron levels. If you are not deficient in these nutrients but your doctor has urged you to use a multivitamin, take the time to read the supplement label to make sure that the multivitamin you choose is free of both copper and iron.

B Vitamins

The B vitamins, sometimes referred to as the vitamin B complex, are best known for helping the body turn food into energy and helping form red blood cells. But many studies have shown that B vitamins also offer benefits to the brain. Research has especially focused on three vitamins in the complex—folic acid (B_9), B_6, and B_{12}—that help lower levels of homocysteine, an amino acid that increases the risk of Alzheimer's disease when present in high levels.

Studies have demonstrated that elevated homocysteine levels are associated with poor brain performance; an increase in the progression from mild cognitive impairment (MCI, Stage 2 of AD) to dementia (Stage 3 of AD); and an increase in the rate of brain shrinkage. It has been suggested that high levels of homocysteine accompanied by low levels of folic acid may make the brain more vulnerable to damage from beta-amyloid, a toxic substance that is a hallmark of AD. For this reason, a study at Oxford University was designed to examine whether lowering homocysteine levels through B supplementation would assist in the fight against AD. Volunteers age seventy and older with a diagnosis of MCI were either given high-dose oral supplements of folic acid, B_6, and B_{12}; or given placebo pills. After two years, the rate of brain shrinkage in people receiving the B vitamins was 30-percent lower than in those taking the placebo, and the effect was greatest in those who had the highest levels of homocysteine. A follow-up study by the same research team showed that B vitamins appear to slow cognitive and clinical decline in people with MCI, especially in those with elevated homocysteine levels, providing benefits in memory and executive function.

It should be noted that B-vitamin supplementation has not clearly been shown to be beneficial for people already in Stage 3 AD. But the Oxford researchers felt that for people not yet diagnosed with dementia, the B vitamins offer a "simple and safe treatment" that may slow brain atrophy.

The B vitamins can be found in most animal proteins—fish, poultry, beef, pork, eggs, and dairy products, especially cheese—as well as in beans, peas, and leafy green vegetables. But after age fifty, some people have trouble absorbing B vitamins from foods. Moreover, the B vitamins are water soluble, meaning that any excess is usually eliminated from the body in urine rather than building up. This makes them relatively safe to use, although B_6 in high amounts (more than 100 mg per day) may be harmful. For this reason, even though further research is necessary to clearly define the role that these nutrients can play in preventing AD, it makes sense for people with elevated homocysteine blood levels to consider taking folic acid, B_6, and B_{12} supplements as a means of protecting the brain. Based on studies, 800 mcg of folic acid, 20 mg of B_6, and 500 mcg of B_{12} are suggested per day. Your doctor may recommend a different dose based on blood tests.

It is important to note that in the studies discussed above, the beneficial effect of B vitamins on the brain was observed only in subjects with high omega-3 fatty acid blood levels. As such, it is clear that these important nutrients are interrelated, which supports the multimodal approach that we advocate in this book. (See page 171 for a discussion of omega-3 fatty acids.)

Vitamin D₃

Vitamin D is best known for helping your body absorb calcium and thus promoting bone strength and growth. But vitamin D may also help protect your brain against cognitive decline and Alzheimer's disease.

Studies have shown that many Americans—well over 50 percent, in fact!—are deficient in vitamin D. The reasons for this deficiency may include low exposure to the sun, which the body needs to produce vitamin D; a decreased ability to both absorb this nutrient and synthesize it as people age; obesity, since vitamin D "gets stuck" in fat tissue and is not easily released; and an inadequate intake of the foods that contain vitamin D, such as salmon, tuna, mackerel, and vitamin D-fortified dairy products.

Doctors have long known that inadequate vitamin D can cause bones to be soft, but more recently, a myriad of studies have suggested that vitamin D deficiency is also associated with a significantly increased risk of Alzheimer's disease. For instance, a sizeable 2014 study, published in *Neurology* journal, showed that people with extremely low levels of vitamin D are more than twice as likely to develop AD or other forms of dementia than people who have normal vitamin D levels. Although studies have indicated that this vitamin may combat inflammation, fight oxidative stress, and stimulate nerve growth factors, the role that it plays in brain function and cognition is not known and merits further investigation. But since vitamin D deficiency is so common, it is prudent to ask your doctor to assess your blood level of this nutrient, and if your level is low, to take steps to increase it.

One way to boost your vitamin D levels is to spend ten to fifteen minutes in direct sunlight between the hours of 10:00 AM and 3:00 PM. But chances are that if you have been diagnosed with a vitamin

D deficiency, you will be given nutritional supplements of D_3, which is considered the best-absorbed form of this nutrient. Vitamin D is a fat-soluble vitamin, which means that it can accumulate in the body and cause problems if you overdose. The main consequence of vitamin D toxicity is a buildup of blood calcium, which can cause a variety of non-specific symptoms, including loss of appetite, nausea, vomiting, weight loss, and frequent urination. To avoid this, follow your doctor's advice regarding dosage. The usual doses of vitamin D_3 are about 1,000 to 2,000 IU in pill form every day—preferably taken with some dietary fat to aid absorption.

Other Supplements

In addition to vitamins, there are a number of other supplements that may prove beneficial to AD management.

Omega-3 Fatty Acids

In Chapter 3, we encouraged you to get plenty of omega-3 fatty acids through your diet by eating fatty fish, olive oil, nuts, and other omega-3-rich foods. This is important because there is significant evidence that omega-3 fatty acids can help protect against and delay the onset of cognitive decline and/or Alzheimer's disease. These essential nutrients—nutrients that must be supplied by your diet—may even improve or stabilize symptoms in patients with certain types of cognitive impairment, such as age-associated cognitive decline.

A study conducted at the University of California at Los Angeles (UCLA) showed that middle-aged and older adults who regularly consume foods high in omega-3s have a reduced risk of the mental decline that leads to dementia. In contrast, low red blood cell levels of the omega-3 known as DHA (docosahexaenoic acid) are associated with smaller brain volume, lower scores on tests of visual memory and executive functions such as problem solving, and less blood supply to the brain. Of even greater significance was the landmark Multidomain Alzheimer Preventive Trial (MAPT study), presented in 2015 at the Clinical Trials on Alzheimer's Disease meeting and published in 2014 in *The Journal of Prevention of Alzheimer's Disease*. A three-year randomized trial, with subjects age seventy and over, MAPT used a multidomain approach that included nutritional counseling, physical exercise, cognitive stimulation, and supplementation with the omega-3 fatty acid DHA. Control groups used the supplementation alone, the multidomain intervention alone, or a placebo. Using brain imaging studies, investigators found that people with low blood DHA benefited considerably from the multidomain intervention plus DHA (800 mg per day), showing significant improvements in brain metabolism. This was especially true in people who tested positive for the APOE4 gene, and in those who already had deposits of beta-amyloid protein—one of the hallmarks of AD—in their brain. The researchers demonstrated that the multimodal approach plus DHA supplementation slows cognitive decline in older adults.

Although further study of the effects of omega-3s on brain health is needed, and we cannot accurately determine who will respond to fatty acids, we are convinced that these nutrients are generally beneficial—particularly when used as a preventative measure or as a management option in the earliest stage of AD (MCI due to AD). Even if you eat fish regularly, you may benefit from two specific omega-3 fatty acids: docosahexaenoic acid (DHA) and eicosapentaenoic acid (EPA). While omega-3 fish oil supplements are usually well tolerated, be sure to check with your doctor before adding them to your daily routine. They may potentially have a blood-thinning effect and must be used with caution in people who take anticoagulant (blood thinning) medications like Coumadin. In addition, there is (very) limited evidence based on one study that men who have a higher risk of prostate cancer may want to avoid higher doses of DHA. As with any supplement, start with a small amount at first, and gradually increase your dosage over time. For those who have a fish allergy or follow a vegetarian diet, algae-based omega-3s are a good alternative. In fact, one of the main studies that showed benefits for people with age-related cognitive decline used an algae-based DHA supplement.

When shopping for fish oil supplements, look closely at the label to determine how much DHA and EPA is in each capsule, and how many capsules constitute a single "serving." We suggest choosing a brand that has at least 200 to 500 mg of DHA, and 100 to 300 mg of EPA in each capsule. While individual recommendations can differ based on a variety of factors, we recommend starting with one capsule a day with a big meal. After a week, if no side effects occur, increase the dosage to two capsules a day, taken together or split into two doses. As already said, omega-3 supplements are considered safe, but you will want to watch for side effects, which can include cough; difficulty swallowing; dizziness; fast heartbeat; hives, itching or skin rash; puffiness or swelling of the eyelids or around the eyes, face, lips, or tongue; tightness in the chest; or unusual fatigue or weakness.

Cocoa Powder

By now, most people know that cocoa—pure and unsweetened—has been found to provide health benefits, including reduced blood pressure. But did you know that cocoa has also been found to improve cognitive function?

Cocoa contains *flavanols,* natural compounds that are antioxidants. In 2012, an exciting study showed that people with mild cognitive impairment who regularly consumed a specific type of purified cocoa powder with high levels of flavanols saw improvements in their memory function. The subjects also experienced improved blood pressure control and insulin sensitivity. A follow-up study in 2014 using the same formulation focused on people between the ages of sixty-one and eighty-five with no evidence of cognitive dysfunction. The subjects were assigned to one of three flavanol groups, consuming either high, intermediate, or low levels of cocoa flavanols for eight weeks. Cognitive function was assessed before and after the study. Among those subjects who consumed either high or intermediate levels of flavanols, the researchers found significant improvements in overall cognitive function. They also found reduced blood pressure and improved insulin resistance.

It's important to note that most methods of processing cocoa remove many of the flavanols found in the raw plant, and the studies discussed above used CocoaVia unsweetened dark chocolate, which was specifically developed to extract flavanols from the cocoa beans. While further research is necessary, we think that the low risk of side effects make it worthwhile to add cocoa flavanols to your brain-healthy lifestyle—especially if you have mild insulin

Coconut Oil

In Chapter 2 (see page 60), we discussed how medium-chain triglycerides (MCTs)—found in various foods, including coconut oil—can result in the production of ketones even in the absence of carbohydrate restriction. This is important, because many people with Alzheimer's disease have a decreased ability to utilize glucose, which is the brain's primary source of fuel, causing the cells to "starve" and eventually die. By providing ketones, an alternative source of fuel that is "cleaner burning" than glucose, MCTs may help protect the brain from damage.

Some reports suggest that the use of coconut oil may be beneficial in the management of AD. Anecdotally, people have reported that the regular use of coconut oil has resulted in an improvement of cognitive powers in people with dementia. In addition, a study by the University of Oxford suggests that coconut oil provides real albeit short-term cognitive benefits. So far, though, there has not been sufficient scientific research on coconut oil to definitively show that it is beneficial. Moreover, some physicians are cautious about recommending coconut oil because it is high in saturated fats, and because certain hydrogenated forms have trans fats that can cause increases in weight and cholesterol levels. Until further research is done, we cannot recommend the use of coconut oil. However, based on your physician's approval, you may consider adding it to your diet.

If you do choose to try coconut oil, be sure to keep track of any changes in weight and to have laboratory studies before and after starting to monitor factors like cholesterol. Also pick a nonhydrogenated form of oil that contains no trans fats, and start with small amounts. The optimal dosage is not yet known, but it is known that taking a large amount of the oil right away can lead to disagreeable side effects, including diarrhea, stomach cramping, bloating, nausea, and vomiting. Individuals with a history of bleeding or inflammatory diseases in the gastrointestinal tract need to be especially cautious about using coconut oil. Note that due to the high fat content of this food, you will need to decrease the rest of your fat intake to avoid gaining weight and straying from the brain-healthy principles of the APT Diet. While using coconut oil, it is a good idea to reduce portion sizes and stick to an active exercise regimen.

resistance, with or without mild memory loss. Note that we're not giving you carte blanche to gorge on dark chocolate! Dark chocolate certainly includes some flavanols, but it usually provides lots of saturated fat and sugar, too. Instead, if you choose not to use CocoaVia, look for unsweetened cocoa powder that is as pure as possible and has not been processed through the Dutch method, which reduces the content of flavanols. Stir 1 or 2 teaspoons into coffee, a smoothie, or yogurt. If the results are too bitter for your taste, add a little natural sweetener, such as agave, which is low-glycemic. We recommend starting slowly with about 150 mg of cocoa flavanols per day. After a week, if the cocoa has been well tolerated, increase the amount to about 375 mg per day.

While this supplement is generally well tolerated, cocoa contains caffeine, and consuming large amounts may cause some caffeine-related effects like sleeplessness, nervousness, a fast heart rate, or increased urination. Cocoa can on occasion also cause a variety of complaints such as allergic skin reactions, headache, constipation, nausea, and gas.

Curcumin

Curcumin is a natural component of the spice turmeric, which has been used in India and other South Asian countries for centuries. Now, there is evidence that a diet rich in curcumin may have protective effects on the brain and reduce the risk of Alzheimer's disease, as well as a variety of other conditions.

Curcumin was investigated as a possible AD treatment because of its anti-inflammatory and antioxidant properties. Epidemiological studies have shown that people who consume turmeric often have a lower incidence of AD than people who do not eat turmeric. However, when it comes to AD treatment, a recent study showed that curcumin supplementation was not effective, which was most likely related to the supplement not being adequately absorbed by the body.

At this time, we believe that the best way to benefit from curcumin's brain-protective properties is to use the spice turmeric in your home-cooked meals, along with some brain-healthy fat to aid absorption. The therapeutic use of curcumin seems promising, perhaps more for AD prevention than treatment. Further research is necessary to clarify the most optimal route of administration, preparation, and dosage.

If you decide to use curcumin supplements, however, be aware that curcumin may strengthen the effects of blood thinners such as Coumadin; may interfere with the action of medications that reduce stomach acid, such as Tagamet; and may strengthen the effects of diabetes medications. For that reason, you should not use curcumin in supplement form without first talking to your physician.

Resveratrol

Resveratrol is a unique phytonutrient (plant chemical) with antioxidant properties. It is found in red and purple grapes, cranberries, blueberries, peanuts, pistachio nuts, and cocoa powder, and is especially abundant in grape skins. For this reason, many people are familiar with it as one of the substances that makes wine "healthy."

While animal studies have shown that resveratrol may delay age-related cognitive decline, data are more limited when it comes to humans with AD and the use of resveratrol for AD prevention. One recent study of 23 people without memory loss found that supplementation with 200 mg of resveratrol each day improved memory function. Using neuroimaging studies, researchers discovered that the function of the memory centers of the brain also improved. A study of 119 people with mild to moderate AD showed that higher doses of synthetically produced purified resveratrol appeared to stabilize levels of beta-amyloid after a year, and were safe and well tolerated. Other studies using higher doses (2,000 mg per day) have also shown intriguing results. Yet further research with larger numbers of people is necessary to clarify the relationship between resveratrol and AD prevention and treatment.

If you want to increase the resveratrol in your diet, consider adding foods that are rich in this substance. Enjoy a small glass of red wine each day, and when planning meals and snacks, include blueberries, pistachio nuts, and cocoa—all of which are recommended on the Alzheimer's Prevention and Treatment Diet. If you prefer supplements, start with about 100 mg a day, and increase if tolerated to a maximum of 500 to 1,000 mg a day. Resveratrol side effects have been reported only anecdotally. At low doses, side effects have included

Additional Supplements Being Researched

There are a number of different supplements that are currently being investigated for their use in Alzheimer's Disease prevention and treatment. These include:

- Alpha-lipoic acid
- Ashwagandha
- Coconut oil (see the inset on page 174)
- Fullerene C_{60}
- Carnitine

- Fisetin
- Lithium
- Magnesium
- Melatonin
- Vitamin C
- Vitamin E

Because the research on these substances is still either conflicting or very limited, we are reluctant to recommend any of them at this time. Yet, in some cases—for example, when a person with a family history of AD is having trouble falling asleep—a supplement like melatonin may be a therapeutic option. (See page 207 of Chapter 7 for information on using melatonin.) If you are interested in trying the alternative supplements mentioned above, talk with your doctor to see if any are viable options for you.

In addition, we'd like to note that some supplements have been researched more extensively and found to be generally ineffective at treating or preventing Alzheimer's disease. These include ginkgo biloba and coenzyme Q_{10} (CoQ_{10}). As such, we do not recommend taking these supplements.

New information on the effects of dietary supplements on cognitive function, dementia, and Alzheimer's disease is always emerging. For an up-to-date overview of current research, we encourage you to visit the websites of the National Center for Complementary and Integrative Health's and the Alzheimer's Drug Discovery Foundation. (See page 234 of Resources.)

stomach cramps, diarrhea, and decreased appetite. At higher doses, arthritis pain, jittery feelings, and tendonitis have occurred. The supplement can also slow blood clotting, so it's important to get approval from your physician before starting resveratrol supplementation.

It's important to note that the recommendations made above are general—that is, we've provided information on supplements that we believe *may* be helpful to the population at large. As the field of nutrigenomics develops, scientists will develop a better sense of how an individual's genetic profile affects his or her capacity to respond to specific nutritional or supplementary approaches. (See page 61 for a discussion of nutrigenomics.) In his own practice, Dr. Isaacson has already begun to use genetic testing in order to tailor his treatments to his patients' unique genes and needs. Unfortunately, genetic testing is new, and individualized treatment regimens are not yet obtainable for the majority of Americans today. Until these approaches are more common, we encourage you to use the information provided above as a guide to supplementing your Alzheimer's Prevention and Treatment Diet.

EXERCISE

As discussed in Chapter 5 (see page 112), exercise is one of the best things you can do to support your cognitive health. Studies almost universally suggest that physical activity can help protect the brain and delay the development of Alzheimer's disease in ways that no drug or nutritional supplement can. Physical inactivity, on the other hand, is increasingly seen as a potential risk factor for AD, raising the likelihood of developing this disease. According to one estimate, over 20 percent of all AD cases in the United States may be attributed to physical inactivity.

How does exercise help your brain? As explained in Chapter 5, exercise increases blood flow to the brain and body and reduces the risk factors for cognitive decline, including high cholesterol, high blood pressure, and diabetes. Physical activity also appears to benefit the hippocampus, your brain's memory center. In older adults, the hippocampus atrophies, or shrinks, over time as part of the normal aging process. In patients with Alzheimer's disease, the hippocampus shrinks more dramatically, which helps explain why memory loss is so pronounced in people with AD. Research indicates that exercise increases activity levels in the hippocampus and may prevent or lessen deterioration of the hippocampus. Exercise may even increase the size of the hippocampus, potentially reversing the aging process. In a study conducted by Dr. Kirk Erickson of the University of Pittsburgh and Dr. Arthur Kramer of the University of Illinois, older adults with no dementia experienced an average 2-percent increase in hippocampus volume after a year of regular aerobic exercise (walking on a track). As a point of reference, a control group of similar adults who did not participate in an exercise regimen showed an average 1.5-percent *decrease* in hippocampus volume over the same time period.

Animal studies have suggested that exercise may increase the size of the hippocampus by raising levels of *brain-derived neurotrophic factor (BDNF)*. BDNF is a protein that encourages the growth and maintenance of brain cells. It also seems to promote neuroplasticity, or the capacity to form new connections between brain cells. Accordingly, higher levels of BDNF are associated with both better memory retention and better learning.

As with other interventions discussed in this book, some people will see greater improvements in memory and brain function than others as a result of exercise, and genetics may play a role in determining how extensively exercise benefits different people. For example, in people who have the APOE4 gene, exercise appears to be particularly effective in reducing amyloid levels in the brain. No matter who you are and what your genetic profile is, however, exercise is still one of the best ways to protect and strengthen brain health. It improves memory and executive function—the so-called higher-order thinking skills involved in planning and performing specific tasks—and may enhance your capacity to learn. With this compelling evidence in mind, we recommend that everybody engage in regular physical activity to either prevent or treat Alzheimer's disease.

What kind of exercise is best, and how much should you get? Some studies have shown that cardiovascular exercise—also called cardio or aerobic exercise—provides the most significant benefits to brain function by getting your heart pumping and your blood circulating. *Cardiovascular exercise* is any exercise that uses muscle movement to raise heart rate. The Centers for Disease Control and the American College of Sports Medicine both recommend that adults strive to engage in moderate- or vigorous-intensity cardio activity. Moderate-intensity cardio activity is defined as exercise that raises your heart rate and makes you break a bit of a sweat. If you can talk but not sing while exercising, your exertion level is considered moderate. Vigorous-intensity physical activity raises your heart rate and sweat level even further—you should not be able to speak more than a few words at a time while exercising at this level. Moderate-intensity activities include brisk walking, riding a bicycle at less than ten miles per hour, doubles tennis, ballroom dancing, and most gardening. Vigorous-intensity activities include jogging or running, swimming laps, singles tennis, and biking at ten miles per hour or faster. (For lists of both cardiovascular and resistance exercises, turn to the inset on page 182.)

For many people, though, resistance training—also known as weight training and weight/resistance training—may be especially important. *Resistance training* includes any exercise that causes muscles to contract against external resistance with the goal of increasing muscle mass, muscle tone, strength, and/or endurance. As you might expect, people who have a higher percentage of body fat may need to focus on resistance training as a means of restoring lost muscle and improving mobility and strength. But resistance training has proven benefits for the brain, as well. One study, conducted by researchers at the University of British Columbia in Vancouver, Canada, showed that when older people with mild cognitive impairment engaged in resistance training twice a week for six months, they performed better than control groups on tests measuring attention, memory, and higher-order brain function.

Before we get into the nitty-gritty of how much exercise you should do and how often you should do it, another type of exercise— a variation of cardio—is worth discussing. Called *interval training*, and also referred to as speed training or speed work, this form of exercise alternates bursts of intense activity with periods of lighter activity. For instance, if your cardio exercise includes brisk walking, you might integrate short (one- or two-minute) bursts of jogging with your normal walking pace. If you're less fit, you might alternative periods of faster walking with your usual leisurely walking. No special equipment or skills are needed. You'll simply be boosting your activity level for only a minute or two at regular intervals. Research has shown that by incorporating interval training with regular training, you can become physically fit in less than half the time normally required.

Generally speaking, the more exercise you do, the better. In Chapter 5, which details our nine-week program of diet and exercise, we recommend that you slowly increase your exercise time over the nine-week period, and that ultimately, you devote 180 minutes a week to exercise, divided into three or four sessions. Strive for roughly a two-to-one ratio of cardio to weight/resistance training. In other words, if you are performing a total of 180 minutes of exercise in a seven-day period, about 120 minutes should be devoted to cardio and about 60 minutes should be devoted to weight/resistance. As you build your exercise time and vary your activities, try to maintain the two-to-one ratio. Mixing in stretching exercises, yoga, pilates, and other types of movement would be valuable. And if you are physically able, consider turning one session of cardio exercise a week into an interval training session.

Although there are great benefits associated with longer, more intense workouts, it's important to understand that even low-intensity activity can be valuable, especially if you've been leading a sedentary lifestyle. One study showed that walking just ten city blocks (about a mile) each day at a pace of twenty to thirty minutes a mile will help preserve brain volume over time. And you don't have to do it all at once; instead, you can fit in extra steps throughout the day. Whether it's taking the stairs instead of the elevator or doing a little cleaning around the house, any physical activity is better than no physical activity.

If it's been a while since you last exercised, talk to your doctor to see if it's safe to proceed with an exercise regimen, and discuss the types of activity that would be most appropriate. If your doctor gives you the go-ahead, begin slowly and develop your capacity over time, increasing both the duration and intensity of your workouts. If mobility issues prevent you from reaching your exercise goal, ask

Suggested Cardiovascular and Weight/Resistance Exercises

If you've already read the discussion of exercise that begins on page 178, you know that both cardiovascular (cardio) and weight/resistance training are necessary for brain health. If you're new to the exercise game, though, you may be wondering which activities fit into the cardio category and which are considered muscle-building activities. The lists below will direct you to some common exercises in each group. As you'll see, you have a range of choices. Some require special equipment, such as a treadmill or weight machine, and some require only a good pair of good running shoes or a space for floor exercises. Several activities—such as water aerobics and elliptical machines—are low-impact, which means they're easier on your back and joints. Ideally, you should get approval from your physician before beginning any exercise program. If you need help in using a piece of equipment or putting together a sound exercise regimen, talk to a fitness instructor.

Cardiovascular Exercises

- Aerobics classes
- Cross-country skiing
- Cycling (regular or stationary bike)
- Dancing
- Elliptical trainers
- Hiking
- Jogging
- Jumping rope
- Rowing (in a boat or on a machine)
- Stair-climbing (on actual stairs or on a machine)
- Swimming
- Tennis
- Walking (outside or on a treadmill)
- Water aerobics

Weight/Resistance Training

- Exercises that use your own body weight, like squats, push-ups, and leg lifts
- Free weights
- Medicine balls (weighted balls)
- Resistance bands
- Weight machines

your physician if physical therapy would be helpful. And if you want to learn more exercise techniques or you find it difficult to maintain your motivation, think about hiring a personal trainer.

Before we leave the subject of exercise, a word or two should be said about cost. Although we've mentioned the relatively expensive option of getting a personal trainer, realize that exercise doesn't have to break the bank. There are lots of activities—like walking, riding a bike, and doing push-ups—that you can perform on your own, without special equipment or instruction. Also, although some gyms have high membership fees, a number of gyms, such as Planet Fitness, are fairly affordable. Many towns also have community and recreation centers that may have open gym times and hold classes like aerobics, yoga, and weight lifting. A similar option is your local YMCA, which generally offers memberships for less than those offered at for-profit gyms. Whether you get your workout at home, on the walking paths of your favorite park, or at a local gym or YMCA, any time and effort you put into physical activity is certain to provide benefits in terms of overall well-being and greater brain health.

INTELLECTUAL ACTIVITY

Study after study has shown an association between mental activity and a lower risk of dementia. In a five-year study of 469 seniors published in *The New England Journal of Medicine*, researchers found that reading, playing board games, and playing a musical instrument all appear to offer protection from dementia. French researchers, too, discovered that activities such as gardening, knitting, and traveling are linked to a lower risk of dementia. Solving crossword puzzles and doing mentally challenging jobs have also been found to lessen the risk of cognitive decline.

Researchers do not know exactly how intellectual activity supports brain health, but it has been suggested that these activities create a rich network of connections between neurons (brain cells), so that if some of these connections break down due to aging or other causes, others take over, preventing or slowing cognitive decline. Whatever the mechanism involved, it seems clear that mental activity offers benefits in terms of brain health.

Research has shown us that some activities are especially helpful in strengthening the brain. For instance, a study at Northwestern University found that people who play a musical instrument often have greater-than-average attention span and memory—both of which are important cognitive powers. Even listening to music is useful, as it causes multiple areas of the brain to become engaged and active, but playing an instrument is more beneficial, as it gives the entire brain a workout. So if you've always wanted to learn how to play the piano or the guitar, start now. Or if you used to sing with your high school choir, look for a community chorus. If you're not interested in playing a musical instrument, simply spend some time each day listening to music. We recommend enjoying stimulating music during the day, and more relaxing or calming music at night.

Another pursuit that is considered a sensible option for more robust brain health is learning a new language. Like playing music, mastering a language gives the brain a workout. It's also been found that people who speak more than one language have better overall cognitive skills compared with those who speak only one. One study even showed that people who are taught a new language experience increased volume of the hippocampus, the memory center of the brain. So consider taking up a new language—or brushing up on a language you once knew. Learn it on your own, or even better, enroll in a class so that you also reap the benefits of socialization. (You'll learn more about that later in the chapter.)

. Below, we've provided some ideas for activities that will keep your mind working—and perhaps even enhance your mental skills over time. Some of these ideas we've already touched on in the above discussion.

- Take up a new hobby or return to one that you enjoyed years ago. Studies have shown that creative hobbies—knitting, embroidering, woodworking, painting, sculpting, and drawing, for instance — are especially helpful in keeping your brain sharp.

- Play a musical instrument, or simply listen to music.

- Learn a new language, preferably, in a group setting.

- Watch thought-provoking movies, including documentaries.

- Read whatever captures your interest, whether books, magazines, or newspapers. (Of course, the more challenging the material, the more likely it is to yield cognitive benefits.)

- Explore a subject of interest by taking a course at a local college or through adult education. Also consider attending lectures provided at local schools, libraries, or community centers.

- Plan a trip to somewhere you've always wanted to go. Read up on your destination, and then explore all that it has to offer. If the preparation for your trip involves learning a new language, all the better.

Keeping your mind active is more than just a good way to stimulate the brain; it's a good way to live your life. By finding interesting pursuits, you will make every day more enjoyable.

SOCIAL ACTIVITY

When you are young and are involved in doing a job and raising a family, a certain amount of social engagement is part of your life. But it can be difficult to stay socially involved as you age. Children grow up and leave the home, you may no longer participate in the work force, and physical limitations may prevent you from getting out as often as you'd like.

There is a very good reason, however, to remain socially active: Research has shown that people who regularly take part in social interaction tend to maintain their brain vitality. In a study conducted by Krister Hakansson in Stockholm, Sweden, researchers studied whether midlife marital status is associated with late-life brain health. It was found that people who live with partners, and therefore have constant interactions with another human being, are 50-percent less likely to experience dementia later in life. Other studies, performed around the world and across the United States, have supported this finding by showing that social interactions—both maintaining existing relationships and developing new ones—may protect memory and delay the onset of dementia. The FINGER study, landmark research that was first discussed in Chapter 4 (see page 93), included socialization in the multimodal approach that was proven to delay cognitive decline. Research has even demonstrated that social engagement may allow you to live longer!

Scientists aren't sure why socialization promotes brain health, although some have suggested that it may stimulate the production of certain hormones that help mediate stress and thus keep the brain from deteriorating. And, like any activity that uses the brain, the "work" of creating and maintaining social relationship may help forge connections between neurons.

So what can you do to become socially active? Here are some suggestions:

- Stay in touch with friends and family—or if you've lost touch over time, make some phone calls and resume contact. Arrange to get together at a restaurant for dinner, invite people over to your home, or make plans to see a movie together. If possible, schedule regular family or group meals and social events.

- Take a class in any subject that appeals to you, from investing to bird watching to making jewelry. As discussed earlier in the chapter, you can find a variety of classes at your local college or through adult education.

- Turn a solitary activity into a group activity. For instance, libraries often host book discussion groups. Knitting shops often have times when people can meet and knit or crochet together. Camera clubs bring together people who enjoy taking photographs. Instead of pursuing these interests alone, share them with others.

- If you're physically able, play a team sport, such as softball. Or join a local bowling team.

- Volunteer your time. Whether you're working on a political campaign, at a hospital, or at a local food bank, you will probably meet like-minded people. Plus, you'll have the satisfaction of giving back to the community.

- Attend a local church, temple, community center, or senior center. There, you will find a host of activities that will put you in touch with other people in your area.

- Visit the website Meetup at www.meetup.com. Designed to bring people together for activities of mutual interest, Meetup offers a range of events in your area. For instance, you'll find book club meetings, bowling nights, movie-and-dining nights, concerts, dances, hikes through parks, and more, with each event hosted by a local group. Because you choose the specific group you "meet up" with—such as baby boomers, mature singles, arts-and-crafts lovers, or tennis enthusiasts—you'll have a good chance of making contact with people you want to know.

If you think that the list above overlaps a bit with the recommended brain-stimulating activities presented on page 184, you're right. Just about any intellectual activity can be turned into a social pursuit, and all social pursuits include a degree of mental stimulation. This is great, as studies have shown that by combining different types of activities—like mental activity and social engagement—you will have a more positive effect on brain health than you would by using one approach alone. And when you add the APT Diet to the mix, you'll be doing even more to safeguard your well-being.

STRESS-REDUCTION TECHNIQUES

For many years, it has been known that chronic stress—stress that continues for a long period of time—contributes to Alzheimer's disease. The studies conducted on this subject have been varied. In Sweden, a group of researchers followed individuals who were age seventy-five and older to examine the effects of job-related stress. They found that those who experienced continued stress on the job had an increased risk of dementia and Alzheimer's. Similarly, an American study showed a link between self-reported stress in the elderly and a higher rate of mental decline. In a study released by the University of California, San Diego School of Medicine, it was found that mice exposed to chronic stress showed cognitive impairment similar to that experienced by humans with AD. In another UC San Diego study, the use of a drug that reduces activity of the brain's stress circuitry was found to prevent the onset of cognitive impairment in mice exposed to stress.

Research has shown that repeated stress hampers the growth of nerve cells and promotes the development of tau tangles and amyloid plaques, both of which are distinctive features of AD. It even leads to shrinkage of the hippocampus, which is the memory center of the brain, and weakening of the prefrontal cortex, which is also important for cognition.

Stress is a part of life, so you can't totally eliminate it. Therefore, it makes sense to learn to manage this condition in order to prevent its brain-altering effects. Physical exercise, adequate sleep, enjoyable activities, and socialization can all help reduce tension. But if you still feel anxious and worried, it may help to try stress-reducing techniques such as progressive muscle relaxation, yoga, visualization, meditation, deep breathing, acupuncture, and biofeedback. Taking periodic vacations is also strongly advised. (Even a three-day weekend can help you to unwind.) For some of these techniques, you can find all the guidance you need through the Internet, books, and CDs. To effectively use others, you will need to contact a qualified professional to instruct you. Considering that stress has been linked to a range of serious disorders, including heart disease, asthma, diabetes, and depression—as well as Alzheimer's—it's clear that addressing chronic feelings of worry should be a priority for anyone who wants to live a long and healthy life.

CONCLUSION

As you can see, there are many different ways to improve your brain health. And, as we've continually emphasized, the best approach to preventing and treating AD is a multimodal approach that combines a brain-healthy diet with supplements, exercise, social and intellectual activity, and stress-reduction techniques. This will give you the strongest possible chance of reducing the likelihood of AD and optimally treating AD.

It is important that you commit to making these lifestyle changes for the long term. Although this may seem like an intimidating prospect, your goal is very achievable if you integrate change slowly. Rome wasn't built in a day, and neither is a healthy lifestyle. Chapter 5 guides you in making small modifications every week—adding healthy foods to your meals, building an exercise program, becoming mentally and socially engaged, and reducing stress. Although we encourage you to follow the guidelines presented in that chapter, you should feel free to modify the pace of change so that it's more comfortable for you. Your goal is not to turn your life upside down, but to slowly and surely replace brain-unhealthy habits with brain-healthy habits that you can follow for a lifetime. Realize that all the efforts you make will bring you invaluable rewards. The most important investment is the investment you make in your health—and in the health of your loved ones!

7.

Managing the Challenges of AD Dementia

As the name suggests, the Alzheimer's Prevention and Treatment Diet presented in Chapter 5 is geared to help protect the brain health and overall well-being of both people who have not yet developed any signs or symptoms of Alzheimer's disease *and* those who have already been diagnosed with the disorder. That being said, as Alzheimer's disease progresses to the middle and later phases of Stage 3—when individuals may become confused, agitated, depressed, or have difficulty feeding themselves—it becomes a challenge to maintain optimal nutrition. In some cases, food cravings or other factors may lead to unhealthy weight gain. Far more commonly, the person with AD experiences unwanted weight loss.

This chapter looks at the challenges to brain-healthy nutrition that often come into play when people experience the symptoms of Alzheimer's disease. It offers suggestions for making mealtimes easier and more pleasant so that individuals with AD are more likely to get the nutrition that they need. It also looks at the way the APT Diet can be modified for people who are experiencing unwanted weight loss or, less commonly, weight gain.

Since diet can be affected—either for better or for worse—by medication, this chapter also looks at the medications that are most commonly prescribed to help manage the symptoms of Alzheimer's disease. Finally, it provides helpful tips and strategies for caregivers and others who have people with AD in their life.

When reading the following pages, always keep in mind that the progression of Alzheimer's disease varies from person to person. For that reason, the strategies that work with one individual may not work with another, and it's important to be flexible in your approach. It's also essential to recognize that while the APT Diet is more likely to provide benefits when it is followed closely, people with AD may be resistant to dietary modifications (or even to following their usual diet). Behavioral and mood changes should be discussed with the treating physician, who may be able to address these issues with proper medication or with nondrug behavioral management techniques. Also be aware that in more advanced AD, people generally have to modify their idea of a healthy diet.

DIETARY ISSUES ASSOCIATED WITH ALZHEIMER'S DISEASE

When people are experiencing mild cognitive impairment (MCI) due to Alzheimer's disease (Stage 2), it may be relatively easy to adhere to the APT Diet and maintain good nutrition and proper weight. But eating difficulties are common among people with AD. As the disease progresses, people often eat less and consequently lose weight. This can happen for a variety of reasons. Many individuals have a diminished appetite. Some simply forget to eat. Some find that their senses of smell and taste fade; don't recognize food, dishes, or utensils when they're put in front of them; or mistakenly eat substances that aren't actually food (such as soap or potting soil used in houseplants). Oral or dental problems such as loose teeth or poorly-fitting dentures can make it physically uncomfortable to chew food, and chronic conditions such as depression, diabetes, digestive issues, and constipation can make patients less interested in eating. Medications for AD or associated health conditions can depress appetite, as well. In Stage 3, people can become more irritable and uncooperative, turning meals into a "battle" rather than a calm time to take in nourishment. And finally, those who have impaired balance, coordination, muscle strength, or motor skills may find it difficult to sit up at the table or feed themselves.

Fortunately, those who care for a person with AD can do a great deal to help insure proper nutrition. First, be sure to make regular doctors' appointments for your loved one. A good personal physician will monitor not only the symptoms related to Alzheimer's disease, but also any other conditions or medications that might affect appetite or weight. It may also be helpful to see a registered dietician, who will be able to help your loved one meet feeding goals and maintain a healthy weight and a balanced diet. If the individual with AD seems to be having trouble swallowing, it may be useful to see a swallowing specialist (most commonly a speech pathologist), who will order certain tests to evaluate the problem and suggest strategies for treating it. For example, the speech pathologist may recommend certain food consistencies, head and neck positions, and/or caregiving strategies.

In addition to seeing a physician, make regular dental appointments. This will help ensure that your loved one's teeth, gums, and dental work stay healthy, allowing her to chew and swallow food without pain or discomfort.

It's useful to keep track of your loved one's eating habits. If you are living with someone who has AD, pay attention to the amounts and types of food eaten and the times at which she tends to get hungry. Also monitor any weight, appetite, and activity changes. If you are not living with the person, have the caregiver keep track of this information for you, as it will help you to identify any new health challenges and, when necessary, enable you to create a better eating schedule and more appropriate meals.

Finally, always keep safety in mind. As already mentioned, people with advanced AD may have trouble swallowing and be at risk of choking. For that reason, basic and more advanced first aid and safety certification, as well as learning the Heimlich maneuver, are advisable for caregivers. Of course, you should always call 911 in the event of any medical or other emergency.

On the next page, you will find some general tips for overcoming appetite and eating difficulties and making mealtimes less frustrating for the person with AD dementia. This will be followed by specific strategies to help people with AD who are unintentionally losing or gaining too much weight.

Minimizing Eating Difficulties for the Person with AD

As you've already read, eating difficulties are common in people with AD, and can range from a lack of appetite to difficulty in performing the actual physical task of eating. The following tips should guide you in making mealtime more pleasant and generally more successful so that your loved one is able get the nutrition she needs.

- Encourage participation and independence—to a point. If your loved one is still capable of feeding herself, great! Similarly, if your loved one is still capable of helping to prepare the meal, set the table, or perform other associated tasks, she will feel more involved and invested in the meal. But safety must be a primary consideration. As a result, we recommend constant supervision of both meal preparation and meal consumption. Avoid giving advanced AD patients responsibilities that may be dangerous, such as using a hot stove or a sharp knife. If you do allow them to perform these tasks, monitor their progress carefully; it's easy for a person with AD to forget that a burner has been left on, for example.

- To the extent that your loved one's current eating habits allow, try to preserve some of the routines that she may have developed over the years. For instance, having foods served in the same way, at the same time, and in the same room each day may go a long way toward getting her to eat regularly and with pleasure.

- Reduce distractions at mealtimes. Distractions can prevent a person with advanced AD from concentrating on eating and only eating. To minimize visual and auditory stimulation, turn off the television and radio and put your cell phone on vibrate. Keep the eating area clean and clear, minimize decorative items and clutter, and make sure that the room is well-lit and at a comfortable temperature. Although sharing a meal can help relax a person with AD, if your family is large and noisy, it may be a better idea to serve the person early and let her join the family mealtime for social reasons.

- Simplify the presentation of the meal so that it's easy for your loved one to see and understand what's been put in front of her.

Avoid fancy, distracting garnishes and other complicated presentations. Similarly, avoid using patterned or multicolored dishes, as they can be confusing to a person with advanced AD. Dishes with a single, solid color—white is good—generally work best.

- Don't overwhelm your loved one with options by offering too many foods at once. You may want to put just a single type of food on the plate at any given time, first some spinach, and then a piece of fish, for instance.

- Make foods easier to eat. If your loved one is still able to feed herself, provide utensils with large, easy-to-grip handles. Try putting meals in bowls, which will contain the food and facilitate self-serving better than flat plates. Serve bite-sized or finger foods— apple slices, sticks of string cheese, chicken pieces, and hard-boiled eggs are examples—that can be eaten with the hands. Or change the consistency of the foods as necessary. For those who have difficulty chewing or swallowing, it may be helpful to purée certain foods to make them smooth. Another option is to simply serve softer foods—yogurt or scrambled eggs, for instance.

- Model appropriate behavior. Sometimes it's helpful to show your loved one how to hold a fork and bring food up to the mouth. After seeing this behavior demonstrated, many people find it easier to imitate it.

- Pay attention to food temperature. Check the temperature of any food you serve. As people with AD age, they lose the ability to gauge food temperature, and can easily burn their mouth if food is too hot. Many beverages are more appealing when served cold; patients may prefer smoothies or protein shakes (see page 149) that have been well chilled or iced. Be aware that warm food which has gotten too cold can also be unappealing.

- If it takes your loved one a long time to finish a meal, consider rewarming part of it. Or present the food in two cycles, serving half of the meal first while keeping the other half warm until she is ready to eat it.

- Encourage your loved one to drink fluids. Dehydration is a com-

mon problem among older people. Because it can increase confusion and lead to constipation and dizziness, make sure she gets
plenty of water throughout the day. Chill drinks to make them
tastier; if necessary, add thickeners to drinks to make them easier
to swallow. If the individual with AD has trouble drinking from a
regular cup, try a kid's cup with a sturdy built-in straw or a sippy
cup. Alternatively, serve fluid-rich foods, like low-glycemic fruits.

- Eat with your loved one. Sharing a meal is a great way to spend
time together and provide an opportunity for her to socialize.
Mealtime should be a positive experience, stimulating the mind of
your loved one and helping to maintain basic skills such as talking
and using a fork or spoon.

- Relax. Let the person with AD take all the time she needs to finish
the meal. If she is still able to feed herself, don't be upset if food
ends up on the floor, the table, or clothing. Your loved one may not
always be able to verbalize feelings, but she may still register your
displeasure or impatience and become distressed.

Dealing with Unwanted Weight Loss

It is fairly common for people with AD, especially in the later stages,
to slowly and steadily lose weight over time. As you've already
learned, this can be caused by a number of factors, many of which—
like changing perceptions of food tastes and aromas, loss of appetite
due to medications, and physical difficulty in eating—result in less
food being eaten. But other factors may come into play, as well. For
instance, there may be an increased expenditure of calories caused by
erratic movements and restless wandering. Emerging research also
shows that weight loss may be a part of the overall metabolic disturbances that can accompany Alzheimer's. In fact, weight loss often
precedes the diagnosis of either MCI or dementia due to AD by several years.

It is advisable to consult with your treating physician to find the
root cause of weight loss, if possible, and to consider management
options, such as the reduction of a medication that may be suppress-
ing appetite. It is also important to determine whether the person

with AD is losing excess body fat versus muscle mass. It is usually fine for someone who is overweight to lose a few pounds, but it is not desirable to lose muscle mass, as this can increase the likelihood of falls. Regular exercise that focuses on resistance/weight training is suggested, if possible. A personal trainer can create a customized plan based on individual needs, and a nutritionist can be valuable in insuring that basic nutritional requirements are being met. (See Chapter 6 for more about exercise.) As already discussed, a speech pathologist or other healthcare professional may be needed in the case of swallowing difficulties.

In addition to the individualized guidance offered by your healthcare team, consider the general tips provided on page 194 for making mealtimes easier and more pleasant. Also bear in mind the following suggestions, which are specifically geared to meet the challenge of unwanted weight loss. Note that when dealing with someone with reduced appetite, you may have to try several strategies to see which one works best.

- If you are following the APT Diet, modify it as needed to provide extra calories. Preferably, add calories in the form of lean protein, like white meat chicken and fish, and foods rich in brain-healthy fats, such as olive oil and nuts. As necessary, provide more generous portions of the most brain-healthy forms of carbohydrates, such as brown rice and whole-wheat bread. For additional calories, you can also swap out nonfat yogurt in favor of low-fat or full-fat yogurt, or replace nonfat cheese with low-fat or regular cheese.

- If necessary, try supplementing regular meals and/or snacks of solid foods with nutritious calorie-rich shakes made with whole, preferably organic grass-fed milk; Greek yogurt; berries, such as blueberries or strawberries; bananas; dark cocoa powder (see page 173); and whey protein (see page 78). This "liquid" meal is especially helpful when people with AD have trouble dealing with solid food.

- Make food as visually appealing as possible. For instance, brightly colored fruits or vegetables in small- to medium-sized portions may be more intriguing than a pile of colorless potatoes.

- Instead of serving three large meals a day, try serving a larger number of nutritious "snacks." Small amounts of food may be less intimidating than a plate piled high with meat and vegetables.

- If possible, increase physical activity through regular exercise—especially resistance/weight training, which can help prevent the loss of muscle mass. At the very least, encourage your loved one to get up and walk around the house or around the block. In addition to being good for brain and overall health, physical activity can increase a person's appetite. Even a little bit of exercise can be beneficial!

- In the earlier list of general mealtime suggestions, we recommended that you eat with your loved one to give her a chance to socialize and to make mealtime a more positive experience. If you can't share the meal, at least take a bite or two of food to prompt her to eat.

- Remember that while we want everyone with Alzheimer's disease to get optimal nutrition at all times, a brain-healthy diet doesn't help a person who won't eat it. Recognize that at some point, your dietary goals are likely to shift focus from brain-healthy foods to *any* foods that your loved one is willing to eat. (See the inset on page 199.)

Dealing with Unwanted Weight Gain

Although unwanted weight gain is less common than weight loss for the person with AD, it is a problem for some people. Usually, excessive weight gain in AD is caused by food cravings, especially cravings for sweets, which are a double threat because they not only introduce too many calories and too much sugar into the diet, but also cause brain-healthy foods to fall by the wayside. Some people with AD simply forget that they have already eaten and add extra meals to their day. And some eat out of the boredom that may be related to their illness. They can no longer participate in the activities that used to fill their time, so they snack or even gorge, usually on unhealthy choices.

When an Individual With Alzheimer's Refuses to Follow the APT Diet

The earlier chapters of this book emphasize the benefits of a brain-healthy diet of lean proteins; nutrient-rich veggies, fruits, and grains; heart-healthy fats; and reduced carbohydrates. This diet, along with other lifestyle changes, can help protect the brain and slow the development of Alzheimer's disease. If Alzheimer's has already started, the APT Diet may slow its progression. In contrast, a diet that doesn't provide good nutrition may cause brain function and overall health to deteriorate at a faster rate.

But as a caregiver, be aware that your dietary goals for your loved one will probably have to change over time. This chapter explains that when a person with Alzheimer's advances to the more moderate and severe phases of the disease, there may a variety of obstacles to following the APT Diet, ranging from loss of appetite to an unwillingness to eat certain foods. As mentioned earlier, a brain-healthy diet doesn't help a person who won't eat it! Malnourishment and being underweight are serious problems for people with advanced AD and should be avoided if possible. As the dementia becomes more severe, it may be necessary to change the diet's focus from brain-healthy eating to eating for adequate nutrition. It's important to avoid turning mealtime into a battle. So if your loved one refuses to eat brain-healthy food or lacks interest in food in general, feed her what she likes best. If she seems to want only a particular kind of meal, such as breakfast, consider serving that meal two or three times a day. Any food—even food not included on the APT Diet—is better than no food at all.

As always, you should consult with the treating physician and/or dietitian to check out possible medical causes of this problem. In addition, the following strategies may help.

- If you're following the APT Diet, modify it as needed to reduce the most brain-unhealthy calories. As far as possible, reduce (or totally eliminate) added sugar, desserts, and fried foods. Choose low-fat dairy products, and limit high-fat foods such as nuts. Remember that even healthy fats are calorie-dense.

- Limit access to sweets and junk foods by keeping them out of the house, locking them away, or disguising them behind plain wrappers.

- Serve nutritious snacks throughout the day, including small portions of sweet (but low-glycemic) fruit, which can help to satisfy sugar cravings. Small nourishing snacks can also be provided for the loved one who has just eaten a meal and wants to eat again directly afterwards. A small plate of vegetables or cut-up fruit can satisfy the desire for more food without adding a lot of extra calories.

- If boredom seems to be the problem, plan appropriate activities that will distract your loved one and help prevent overeating. Activities that burn calories—such as taking a walk, if feasible—are particularly helpful. (Walking can help stimulate the brain and improve mood, too.) But any pursuit that engages the person's interest, such as looking through family photos or singing old familiar songs, may have the added benefit of reducing the overconsumption of foods.

MEDICATIONS

Although as of yet, no medication can cure or stop Alzheimer's disease, a variety of prescription medications are routinely prescribed to reduce AD symptoms. These drugs can provide patients with greater comfort and the ability to remain independent for a longer period of time. In addition, some people with AD can benefit from the use of medications that were not specifically designed for AD but can positively affect either the disorders that may contribute to AD or the behavioral changes associated with Alzheimer's.

Sometimes it may seem that medications work against a sound diet, since possible side effects can include nausea, diarrhea, and loss of appetite. But by treating confusion, improving awareness, and otherwise enhancing the individual's ability to carry on daily activities, medications may also make it possible for the person with AD to follow a healthy diet for a longer period of time. The goal is always to optimize the effectiveness of medication while minimizing potential side effects, including those that can affect nutrition. This can be partly achieved by timing meals and medications wisely so that they work hand in hand.

Medications for Alzheimer's Disease

The FDA-approved medications used in Alzheimer's disease are a critical component of any AD treatment plan, as they can help manage symptoms and can even stabilize or improve cognitive function for a time. But, as mentioned above, they can also cause side effects, some of which can interfere with the objective of following a brain-healthy diet. That's why it's so important to use the medications properly, adjusting the dosage as necessary and timing drug doses with meals when advisable.

The medications prescribed for AD fall into two categories— cholinesterase inhibitors and NMDA antagonists. In some cases, patients take a medication from only one of these two categories, and in other cases, especially later in the disease process, they may be given both a cholinesterase inhibitor and an NMDA antagonist. Table 7.1 provides a quick look at the AD medications now being used, along with their categories, the forms in which they're available, and their most common side effects. The following discussions provide more detailed information about each drug's use.

It's important to note that the information provided below represents the drug protocols recommended by most healthcare providers, but is not meant to replace the specific protocol provided by your treating physician. AD medications should be taken only with the approval, review, and ongoing supervision of a physician, and any adverse reactions should be reported to the physician immediately.

Cholinesterase Inhibitors

The brain's nerve cells, called neurons, communicate with one another by releasing chemicals called *neurotransmitters*. The neurotransmitter acetylcholine is known to play an important role in memory and learning—and is also known to be in abnormally short supply in people with Alzheimer's disease. Moreover, acetylcholine is effective only briefly, and is then destroyed by enzymes called cholin-

Table 7.1 Medications Used to Treat Alzheimer's Disease

Drug Name: Brand/Generic	Drug Type and Use	Available Forms of Drug	Common Side Effects
Aricept (donepezil)	Cholinesterase inhibitor used to treat symptoms of mild, moderate, and severe Alzheimer's disease.	• Tablets • Oral disintegrating tablets	Diarrhea, fatigue, muscle cramps, nausea, vomiting, weight loss.
Exelon (rivastigmine)	Cholinesterase inhibitor used to treat symptoms of mild, moderate, and (in case of patch) severe Alzheimer's disease.	• Capsules • Patch • Oral solution	Decreased appetite, diarrhea, muscle weakness, nausea, vomiting, weight loss.
Namenda (memantine)	NMDA antagonist used to treat symptoms of moderate to severe Alzheimer's disease.	• Tablets • Oral solution • Extended-release capsules (Namenda XR)	Confusion, constipation, diarrhea, dizziness, headache.
Namzaric (memantine/ donepezil)	NMDA antagonist and cholinesterase inhibitor used to treat symptoms of moderate to severe Alzheimer's disease.	• Extended-release capsules	Decreased appetite, diarrhea, dizziness, headache, nausea, vomiting.
Razadyne (galantamine)	Cholinesterase inhibitor used to treat symptoms of mild to moderate Alzheimer's disease.	• Tablets • Oral solution • Extended-release capsules (Razadyne ER)	Decreased appetite, diarrhea, nausea, vomiting, weight loss.

esterases. As the name of this drug category implies, *cholinesterase inhibitors* stop or inhibit this breakdown, slowing the destruction of acetylcholine so that more of it is available for communication between brain cells.

The category of cholinesterase inhibitors includes three medications—Aricept (donepezil), Exelon (rivastigmine), and Razadyne (galantamine)—each of which comes in three progressively higher dose levels. In most cases, the treating physician decides to start one of these medications when a person is diagnosed with mild dementia due to AD. All three of these drugs are FDA-approved to treat mild to moderate dementia due to AD, and Aricept and Exelon are also approved to treat severe dementia due to AD.

Doctors generally start patients at the lowest possible dose and continue that dose for four weeks (or occasionally more) to see whether the drug is tolerated—that is, that there are no significant side effects. Side effects are uncommon at a low dosage level, but may include nausea, vomiting, diarrhea, loss of appetite, and weight loss. (See Table 7.1 for the most common side effects of each drug.) These effects are more likely to occur at higher doses, when medications are taken on an empty stomach, and/or in people with low body weight (less than 110 pounds). To avoid side effects with the oral forms of these medications, it is advisable to take them with a big meal, usually breakfast or lunch (whichever meal is larger), as food can improve tolerability. Since the Exelon capsules need to be taken twice a day, each dose should be taken with a meal—preferably, a substantial breakfast and dinner. Because the rivastigmine in the Exelon patch is absorbed by the body gradually, over a twenty-four-hour period, it is less important to eat a full meal when the patch is placed, although regular healthy meals eaten throughout the day can help minimize side effects.

If any side effects are experienced, the treating physician may advise to skip a few doses and retry the drug again in the future, or to reduce the overall drug dosage—for instance, by taking half of a pill instead of a whole pill—until the negative effects disappear. At that point, the baseline dosage may be tried again. If no side effects occur, after four or more weeks, dosage is often increased to the next level to improve the drug's efficacy. Doctors continue to monitor for side effects, and may reduce the dose if adverse symptoms occur. Depending on the individual patient's response, after a few months at a medium-level dosage with no side effects, or when cognitive decline worsens, doctors may suggest raising the dose. Note that because the risk of side effects increases with higher dosages, patients need to remain in regular contact with their doctors to track any unwanted symptoms. It is also important to note that several medical conditions, such as gastroesophageal reflux disease (GERD), may increase the chance of side effects.

When someone does not tolerate a particular cholinesterase inhibitor, she may be able to tolerate another, so the treating physician may consider switching brands. Doctors may also switch and prescribe another cholinesterase inhibitor if the one currently used seems to be ineffective or the person continues to decline.

For best results, it's important to avoid missing doses of AD medication. Dr. Isaacson has had several individuals who stopped taking their medication for days or weeks and suffered cognitive decline. After restarting the medication, they were not able to return to the same level of cognition they had experienced before stopping. We thus encourage caregivers and patients to work together to ensure that any and all medications are taken on a routine basis and as directed—with a large meal, for instance.

One small study showed that taking the B-vitamin folic acid along with the cholinesterase inhibitor Aricept increases the effectiveness of the Aricept. If Aricept is prescribed, talk to the doctor about the possibility of taking folic acid. When taking folic acid, it advisable to also take B_{12}, as the two nutrients work closely with each other. (For more information about the B vitamins and brain health, see page 168.)

NMDA Antagonists

Glutamate is a major neurotransmitter in the brain, and is responsible for communication between the brain's neurons, memory formation, and learning. It is thought that some of the symptoms of Alzheimer's may be associated with excessive excitation of the NMDA (N-methyl-D-aspartate) receptors, which are the brain's receptors for glutamate. *NMDA antagonists* work by binding to the NMDA receptors and regulating the activity of glutamate for better cognitive function.

Namenda (memantine) is the one drug that acts only as an NMDA antagonist, and it is available in different forms, including extended-release capsules. The medication Namzaric (memantine/ donepezil) combines donepezil, the cholinesterase inhibitor already discussed, with memantine. Both drugs are used to treat moderate to severe dementia due to Alzheimer's.

Namenda is usually started at a low dose and taken once a day. Gradually, the amount is increased by stepping up the strength and taking it twice a day, if tolerated. Side effects are not frequent but can include confusion, constipation, dizziness, diarrhea, or headache. This medication does not need to be taken with food. Namenda XR, the extended-release form of the drug, is taken once daily. The dosage is usually increased slowly until maximum dosage is reached.

The medication Namzaric may be suggested in an effort to reduce the overall number of pills taken each day, since it is a combination drug. However, it is started only after the patient has been stabilized on separate doses of memantine and donepezil. Common side effects include reduced appetite, diarrhea, dizziness, headache, nausea, and vomiting. Since this pill includes donepezil, which can cause side effects if taken on an empty stomach, it is advisable to take Namzaric with a meal.

How Long Are AD Drugs Taken?

Usually, people with Alzheimer's take their AD medications for the duration of their condition, but some physicians may stop these medications toward the end of life. It is important to note that when the decision is made to stop these drugs, it is prudent to slowly reduce doses over time rather than discontinuing use all at once. It is also important to understand that eliminating these medications may lead to a worsening of the person's condition, including behavioral changes, so that any and all changes need to be discussed in detail with the treating physician.

Other Medications Used for the Person with AD

Doctors often prescribe additional medications for Alzheimer's patients, either to manage conditions that may contribute to the progression of AD, or to manage additional symptoms that may occur as AD progresses.

Because cardiovascular disease can increase the pace at which Alzheimer's disease advances, doctors must pay close attention to their patients' heart health. Blood pressure and cholesterol levels should be monitored on a regular basis and treated with appropriate medications as needed. Close monitoring and treatment are also essential when the patient has diabetes, another condition that is associated with Alzheimer's. Interestingly, ongoing trials are now investigating the potential for certain diabetes drugs to have beneficial effects on the Alzheimer's disease process.

Behavioral changes—depression, lack of interest in activities, irritability, and personality changes—are fairly common throughout the course of Alzheimer's. Once a person is already taking one or more of the AD drugs discussed earlier, many specialists recommend using certain medications that are FDA-approved for depression and, at lower doses, have also been shown to help relieve other troubling behaviors, like agitation. The drugs that are most commonly used for these purposes belong to a class called *selective serotonin reuptake inhibitors,* or *SSRIs,* which work by increasing concentrations in the brain of the neurotransmitter serotonin, the so-called happiness hormone. The SSRI that has been most studied is Celexa (citalopram). Lexapro (escitalopram), another medication in this category, is also used. Note that neither of these drugs is FDA-approved for treating AD itself, and as such, the doctor needs to review the potential risks and benefits of this therapy before prescribing it for someone with Alzheimer's. The most common side effects of SSRIs include nausea, nervousness or restlessness, dizziness, drowsiness, insomnia, and headache, as well as weight gain or loss. It is advisable to maintain lower doses of Celexa, as higher doses may lead to abnormal heart rhythms.

Another strategy that has recently been studied involves the drug Nuedexta, which is a combination of dextromethorphan and quinidine. While at this time, Nuedexta is not FDA-approved specifically for treating AD patients, it is used to manage the rare but occasional symptom called *pseudobulbar affect,* or *PBA,* which is characterized by uncontrollable, extended episodes of crying and/or laughing. The most common side effects of Nuedexta include diarrhea, dizziness, coughing, vomiting, weakness, swelling of feet and ankles, and gas.

When the drugs already discussed do not help manage some of the more severe behavioral symptoms of AD, such as agitation and aggression, some doctors prescribe a class of medications called *antipsychotics*, which include Seroquel (quetiapine), Risperdal (risperidone), and Zyprexa (olanzapine). Note that these drugs bear what is called a "black box" warning, meaning that the FDA has clearly stated that they may increase the likelihood of harmful medical outcomes, including death. That being said, antipsychotics, which are usually started in low doses, can be helpful in certain situations. The risks and benefits should be described in detail by the treating physician, and because side effects can be serious—and may include the worsening of dementia, shaking and unsteadiness, and an increased risk of blood clots and stroke—any antipsychotic should be used only under constant supervision and must be regularly reviewed.

Be aware that not all behavioral symptoms experienced by people with Alzheimer's are necessarily the result of AD. Instead, coexisting medical illnesses may be the actual cause. For example, when a person with AD gets a urinary tract infection, it may manifest itself as a behavioral change such as confusion, agitation, or sleepiness. That's why it's so important to report any behavioral problems immediately and to look for possible underlying conditions before you choose a treatment.

Another common AD-related issue that may require medication is insomnia. As Alzheimer's progresses, many people sleep only for short periods of time, and may actually get more sleep during the day than at night, when they may awaken frequently. As we first discussed on page 113, whenever possible, disruptions of the sleep/wake cycle should be handled without medication. Most doctors prefer to avoid using certain sedative medications like the benzodiazepines—Valium (diazepam), Xanax (alprazolam), and Ativan (lorazepam), for instance—as well as sedative-hypnotics such as Ambien (zolpidem). While these drugs may help initially, in most cases, they are poor long-term solutions. Instead, many doctors suggest better-tolerated alternatives, such as the supplement melatonin or the antidepressant trazodone, which is known for its sleep-promoting effects. As with all of the medications discussed above, the strategy of "start low, go slow" is best. As an example, it is usually suggested that the patient start taking melatonin in .5-mg or 1-mg doses about fifteen to twenty minutes before bedtime. The dose can then slowly be increased to about 3 mg if approved by the treating physician. If this is not helpful, trazodone may be taken about thirty minutes before bedtime, again starting with a low dose. As with any and all therapies, these options should be discussed and approved by the physician before your loved one begins treatment, and any side effects should be noted and reported.

ADVICE FOR CAREGIVERS

Caring for a person with Alzheimer's can be a challenging task. It can be difficult to see someone you love lose memory, communication, and motor skills, or to undergo personality or behavior changes. It can be even harder to be the primary caregiver for a person whose condition worsens over time. In addition to being emotionally draining, tending to someone with AD requires large investments of time, energy, and money. On the other hand, because only limited medical treatments are now available for people with AD, it is your efforts that will make the most significant difference in your loved one's daily life.

The first step in becoming a good caregiver for someone with AD is to educate yourself and any family members or friends who spend time with the person. Since you've gotten this far in the book, you already have a pretty good foundation of knowledge about the disease, but it never hurts to have more information. Online, there are a number of dedicated and reliable education sites on AD; some even offer free classes for caregivers. You'll find a list of these resources beginning on page 229. By learning as much as you can about the disease—its stages, its treatments, effective ways to manage difficult behavior, and more—you will be better prepared to handle the many new tasks and responsibilities that come with caring for a person with AD. As your knowledge grows, you'll also become more confident in your abilities.

Because caregiving can be very stressful, it's critical that you have outlets for any frustration, anger, or sadness you may feel, and that you take steps to safeguard your physical and emotional health. Don't forget, your needs are just as important as your loved one's! To maintain your own well-being, keep these tips in mind:

- **Maintain a strong support network.** Friends and family can help lighten the burden, both in terms of actual responsibilities—running errands, preparing meals, minding your loved one, etc.—and in terms of the emotional and psychological toll those responsibilities sometimes take. Don't be afraid to ask them for help.

- **Talk it out.** Many people find it helpful to talk about their experiences of caring for a parent, spouse, or relative with AD. If you don't feel comfortable discussing your situation with family or friends, consider seeing a therapist or social worker, or take part in a support group for relatives of AD patients. Support groups can also provide helpful insights and advice on caring for people with Alzheimer's. Even if the person you talk to can't provide solutions to your problems, the simple act of sharing your feelings may be therapeutic.

- **Manage your stress.** Taking care of a person with AD may be one of the most stress-producing tasks you'll ever undertake. To combat this stress, you may need to try some new activities or techniques or to be more diligent about using those techniques that you already practice. Exercise, yoga, and meditation are three great ways to channel your energy, calm your mind, and boost your mood. If you choose exercise, aim for at least thirty minutes a day, but if that proves too difficult, try to fit in several ten-minute sessions.

- **Don't forget to play.** A daily dose or two of fun is not just enjoyable—it is also good medicine. If your loved one is in an early stage of Alzheimer's, you may be able to include her in piecing together jigsaw puzzles, playing simple board games, taking walks, or planting a small flower garden. As the AD progresses, be sure to build in some fun time for yourself by playing with a pet, practicing your golf swing, doing crossword puzzles, knitting, sketching—whatever interests you. Remember that the Internet offers lots of activities, such as online Scrabble tournaments, that may be easy to play when you're "on the job."

- **Take care of your own health.** When you're busy caring for the needs of a loved one, it's easy to neglect your own health. But if

The Ten Warning Signs
of Caregiver Stress and Burnout

Caring for someone with Alzheimer's can be highly stressful, emotionally draining, and physically exhausting. On pages 209 to 211, we present tips for taking care of yourself while you take care of your loved one. Nevertheless, it's easy to become overwhelmed, which is why it's been estimated that 30 to 40 percent of dementia caregivers experience unhealthy levels of stress and depression. If you experience any of the following symptoms on a regular basis, recognize them as the signs of caregiver stress or burnout, and take the time to talk to your doctor so that you can get the help you need.

1. Denial about the disease and its effect on your loved one. ("I think that Dad is getting better.")

2. Anger at the person with AD, at yourself, or at the people around you. ("Why does she keep asking me that same question?!")

3. Withdrawing socially from friends, family members, and activities that you used to find pleasurable.

4. Anxiety about your ability to deal with what lies ahead.

5. Depression, with feelings of sadness and hopelessness.

6. Exhaustion that makes it difficult or impossible to take care of your daily tasks.

7. Sleeplessness caused by never-ending worries.

8. Irritability that leads to emotional behavior and outbursts.

9. An inability to concentrate on and complete tasks.

10. Health problems, including continually feeling unwell, unintended weight loss or gain, frequent colds or other illnesses, and chronic disorders such as high blood pressure and headache.

you do, you will end up harming not only yourself but also the loved one for whom you're caring. So be sure to visit your doctor for regular checkups, and if you find yourself experiencing caregiver stress (see the inset on page 210), contact your doctor or the Alzheimer's Foundation for help.

- **Seek outside help.** It may not be possible or advisable for you to be the sole care provider for your loved one, and you may not be able to get family and friends to help out. If that's the case, look elsewhere for practical assistance. Home health care, adult day care, respite care, a visiting nurse, and hospice services can help you take care of your loved one, whether it's just for a few hours or as a more long-term arrangement. In some areas, volunteer organizations may be able to give you some support. Ask your loved one's doctor for local recommendations, and if possible, compare providers online at Home Health Compare, a service offered by Medicare. (See page 234 of the Resources section.)

Throughout the journey of caring for someone with Alzheimer's, be kind to yourself and to your loved one. As the National Institute on Aging says, it's important to remember that it's the disease, and not the person with AD, that's causing memory loss and personality changes. As AD progresses, the ability of your loved one to show gratitude for your hours of attention will fade, which may make your work seem thankless. For many people, though, the time spent caring for someone with Alzheimer's—and making a positive difference in their life—offers invaluable rewards.

CONCLUSION

As Alzheimer's disease progresses, it becomes a challenge to maintain good nutrition, which is the focus of this book. Nevertheless, as this chapter has shown, there are many strategies that can help people with AD avoid unintentional weight loss or gain and get the nourishment they need for better overall health and greater protection of the brain. This chapter has also explained how medications—both those intended specifically for people with AD and those designed to treat other problems—can be effectively used in AD care, and can be timed and adjusted to help promote a sound diet. Finally, because taking care of a loved one with AD is such a demanding task, this chapter provides invaluable advice for caregivers so that they can maintain their own health even as they attend the needs of another. Adequate care and support for both the patient and the caregiver can go a long way toward maximizing the quality of life for all involved.

Conclusion

Research has shown that diet is one of the greatest weapons available to protect and defend your brain against Alzheimer's disease. Based on current studies, *The Alzheimer's Prevention and Treatment Diet* is your step-by-step guide to selecting foods and creating meal plans that can help reduce the risk for AD, and may help slow its progress if it has already developed. It also suggests specific brain-enhancing activities, from physical exercise to social and intellectual engagement, enabling you to take a multifaceted approach to brain health.

Having worked with thousands of patients—both those who have normal cognitive health and those who are in the early stages of Alzheimer's—we know that this approach can be effective. We also know that it requires commitment. Our diet is designed to ease you into a brain-healthy lifestyle, but only you can take that first step toward improving your brain health by making incremental changes over time, and only you can stick with the diet as you face the challenges of everyday life. As you follow the program, this book will continue to support you with proven strategies and tactics that have helped many others maintain a brain-healthy lifestyle.

We still have much to learn about Alzheimer's disease, and our approach to preventing and managing this disorder will be fine-tuned over time, as research tells us more about the disorder's causes and development. As you've learned in this book, one of the most promising keys to AD therapy appears to be nutrigenomics, the field of science that studies the relationship between the foods we eat and our genetic makeup. As progress is made in this field, we are sure to increase our knowledge about how genetic variations help determine an individual's response to specific nutrients and foods, how food influences genetic expression, and how genes regulate nutritional requirements. This may enable us to offer more personalized disease treatment and prevention—not just for Alzheimer's disease, but also for a myriad of other conditions.

Throughout the pages of this book, we have encouraged you to visit Alzheimer's Universe (www.AlzU.org), which provides information about Alzheimer's, offers lessons and activities that will help you optimize your approach to brain health, and allows you to track your progress as you follow the APT Diet. You can rely on this site to continue to provide current information about AD and its treatment. We also urge you to explore the organizations listed in the Resources section (see page 229), many of which feature continually updated discussions of Alzheimer's. Moreover, as progress is made in AD research, future editions of this book will be revised to reflect breakthroughs in prevention and management.

Although we look forward to gaining more insight into AD, the fact is that *right now* is the perfect time to start adopting a brain-healthy way of life. Both your diet and your lifestyle are within your control, and we know that by making simple changes, you can protect and even enhance your cognitive health. Having read this book, you are well prepared to make informed decisions about the food you eat and about the daily activities that can significantly enhance your well-being—now and for a lifetime. We wish you all the best.

Glossary

Occasionally, this book uses terms that are common in discussions of Alzheimer's disease and/or nutrition, but may not be completely familiar to you. You may also hear these terms when working with doctors, dieticians, and other healthcare professionals. To help you better understand Alzheimer's literature and participate in discussions with your physician, definitions are provided below for words that that are often used by those who diagnose and treat AD and those who work in the field of nutrition. All terms that appear in *italic type* are also defined within the glossary.

aerobic exercise. See *cardiovascular exercise.*

age-associated cognitive decline. Cognitive changes attributed to aging rather than a disorder such as *Alzheimer's disease.*

age-related memory loss. A form of *age-associated cognitive decline* that primarily affects memory, and does not significantly affect other cognitive abilities.

agnosia. The loss of the ability to recognize objects, faces, voices, or places.

Alzheimer's disease (AD). A slowly progressing degenerative disease that attacks the *neurons,* or nerve cells. This results in the gradual loss of memory, thinking, and language skills, and causes changes in behavior.

amino acids. The building blocks of *proteins.* There are twenty common amino acids. Eleven of them can be made by the body and are considered nonessential because they don't have to be supplied by the diet. The nine amino acids that must be supplied by the diet are considered essential.

amyloid plaques. See *beta-amyloid plaques.*

antipsychotics. A class of medications that were created to treat patients with psychotic disorders, but are sometimes used to manage the more severe behavioral symptoms of *Alzheimer's disease,* such as agitation and aggression. (Note that these drugs are not FDA-approved for these purposes.) This class of medications includes Risperdal (risperidone), Zyprexa (olanzapine), and Seroquel (quetiapine), among others. Because antipsychotics bring with them a risk of harmful and even fatal side effects, they should be used only when other drug therapies have failed to control symptoms.

aphasia. The loss of the ability to communicate, whether through speech or through writing, as well as to understand verbal and written language.

APOE gene. See *apolipoprotein epsilon gene.*

apolipoprotein epsilon gene. Generally referred to as APOE, the gene whose main job is to help regulate cholesterol transport and metabolism. There are three different forms of this gene: APOE2, APOE3, and APOE4. People who inherit APOE4 have a higher risk of developing *Alzheimer's disease.*

apraxia. The loss of the ability to perform purposeful movements and tasks, such as combing hair, brushing teeth, or driving.

beta-amyloid plaques. Clumps of a protein called beta-amyloid that form in the brain in the spaces between the nerve cells (*neurons*), preventing them from communicating with one another and eventually leading to nerve cell death. These plaques are considered one of the hallmarks of *Alzheimer's disease.*

biomarkers. A measureable substance, structure, or process in the body that indicates the presence or outcome of a disease.

blood sugar. The *glucose* (sugar) found in the blood, also called blood glucose.

blood-brain barrier. A complex network of special cells that separate the blood circulating throughout the body from the fluids that nourish and surround the brain. The barrier helps keep harmful chemicals out and allows essential substances like glucose to come in.

body composition analysis. A test that measures the proportions of the components of a person's body, including fat, water, and muscle.

body mass index (BMI). A measure of body fat based on height and weight that applies to adult men and women.

brain plasticity. See *neuroplasticity.*

brain-derived neurotrophic factor (BDNF). A protein that encourages the growth and maintenance of brain cells. BDNF also seems to promote *neuroplasticity,* or the capacity to form new connections between brain cells.

caloric restriction. The practice of limiting calorie intake. Caloric restriction has been found to lower the risk for cardiovascular disease, help lower *insulin* levels, lower inflammatory markers, lower blood pressure, and help protect against *Alzheimer's disease.*

carbohydrates. One of the *macronutrients,* present in food in the form of starch, sugar, and fiber. Produced by plants during the process of photosynthesis, carbohydrates are the body's primary source of energy. The carbohydrates that provide energy are divided into two groups—simple carbohydrates and complex carbohydrates. Simple carbohydrates, usually called sugars, have simple chemical structures that quickly break down into glucose when they're consumed. They occur naturally in fruits, vegetables, and dairy products. Complex carbohydrates, often called starches, have more complex chemical structures that are broken down more slowly into glucose when they're consumed. They are found in whole grains, legumes, and certain vegetables. A third group of carbohydrates, fiber—found in whole grains, fruits, vegetables, beans, nuts, and seeds—cannot be digested and therefore cannot be broken down into glucose. Fiber does, however, help regulate the body's use of sugars.

cardiovascular exercise. Also called cardio exercise and aerobic exercise, any exercise that uses muscle movement over time to raise heart rate.

caregiver stress. Also called caregiver syndrome and caregiver burn-out, a condition that can result from caring for someone who is chronically ill. It is especially common when the patient has behavioral difficulties such as dementia. Symptoms of caregiver stress can include fatigue, stress, anxiety, exhaustion, depression, and feelings of guilt.

celiac disease. An autoimmune disorder that causes inflammation and damage to the small intestine when *gluten* is consumed.

cholesterol. A waxy substance, found in all cells, that can be made by the body or consumed in various foods, such as meat, fish, eggs, butter, cheese, and milk. There are two types of cholesterol. Low-density lipoprotein (LDL) cholesterol, sometimes called "bad" cholesterol, carries cholesterol away from the liver into the bloodstream, where it can stick to and clog blood vessels. High-density lipoprotein (HDL) cholesterol, sometimes called "good" cholesterol, picks up excess cholesterol in the blood and carries it back to the liver, where it is broken down.

cholinesterase inhibitors. The largest category of medications prescribed to manage the symptoms of *Alzheimer's disease*. Cholinesterase inhibitors work by inhibiting the breakdown of the *neurotransmitter* acetylcholine, so that more is available in the brain to facilitate memory and learning. This class of medications includes Aricept (donepezil), Exelon (rivastigmine), and Razadyne (galantamine).

cognitive decline. A deterioration in cognitive functions characterized by increasing difficulties with memory, information processing, language, and other functions related to knowing and perceiving. Cognitive decline can be caused by the aging process or by a variety of medical conditions, including *Alzheimer's disease*.

cognitive reserve. The ability of an individual to experience progressive brain pathology, such as *Alzheimer's disease*, without showing the usual severity of clinical symptoms of the disease. This reserve is sometimes described as a backup system for the brain that compensates for any brain damage or shrinkage that occurs in excess of the natural aging process.

cognitive skills. Brain-based skills needed to understand and function in the world. These skills include memory, attention (focus), comprehension, flexibility (the ability to think about several concepts at once and look at them from different perspectives), visual-spatial skills, application of concepts to solve problems, analysis of information, synthesis of new ideas by putting parts of old ideas together, and evaluation of information.

complete protein. A protein source (such as poultry) that contains all nine of the *essential amino acids,* which must be provided by the diet to enable the body to build cells, muscles, and organs.

complex carbohydrates. See *carbohydrates.*

cruciferous vegetables. Members of the Brassicacea family (cabbage family), including (but not limited to) broccoli, Brussels sprouts, cabbage, cauliflower, and radishes.

dementia. A general term used to describe a decline in memory or other cognitive skills that are sufficiently severe to affect an individual's ability to perform everyday tasks. *Alzheimer's disease* is the most common cause of dementia.

dementia due to AD. Stage 3 of *Alzheimer's disease,* characterized by memory loss and other cognitive impairments that interfere with the activities of daily living.

diabetes. A metabolic disease that results in too much *glucose* in the blood. In type 1 diabetes, the pancreas produces little or no *insulin,* the hormone needed to allow glucose to enter the body's cells to create energy. In type 2 diabetes—the most common form of the disorder—the body is not able to use insulin properly (a condition called *insulin resistance*) and also not able to produce enough insulin to compensate for the body's resistance.

diabetic ketoacidosis. See *ketoacidosis.*

dietary pattern. A specific style of eating, usually referred to as a diet.

early-onset Alzheimer's disease. Also called younger-onset Alzheimer's disease, a form of AD that affects people younger than sixty-five years of age. Because certain forms of early-onset Alzheimer's are inherited, it may also be called familial Alzheimer's disease.

essential amino acids. The nine *amino acids* that must be provided by the diet to enable the body to create various structures, including cells, muscles, and organs.

essential fatty acids. Forms of *polyunsaturated fats* that your body needs but can't manufacture on its own. These fats are termed "essential" because they have to be included in the diet. Included among these fats are omega-3 and omega-6 fatty acids, which have many health benefits and are believed to reduce the risk of heart disease, stroke, cancer, and Alzheimer's disease. Good sources of omega-3 fatty acids include salmon, tuna, sardines, mackerel, walnuts, flaxseed, and canola and soybean oil. Good sources of omega-6 fatty acids include safflower oil, grapeseed oil, sunflower oil, and soybean oil. The modern diet tends to provide more omega-6 fatty acids than omega-3 fatty acids.

executive function. The high-level set of mental skills that allow you to coordinate other cognitive skills in order to organize, plan, and execute tasks, including everyday activities like food shopping. Paying attention, planning, sequencing, solving problems, abstract thinking, and selecting relevant sensory information are all part of executive function.

familial Alzheimer's disease. See *early-onset Alzheimer's disease.*

fat. One of the macronutrients, used as a fuel source and to perform various functions in the body, such as the control of cholesterol. Dietary fat comes in many varieties, including *saturated, monounsaturated, polyunsaturated,* and *trans.* Also, a normal constituent of the human body that stores extra calories and also helps insulate the body. When the body has used up calories from carbohydrates, it begins to burn fat for the energy it needs to function.

fiber. See *carbohydrates.*

flavanol. A naturally occurring compound with strong antioxidant abilities found in various plants, including apples, grapes, tea, cocoa, and cherries.

functional plasticity. See *neuroplasticity.*

glucose. The main sugar that the body makes from food and uses to provide energy for all of its activities.

glucose hypometabolism. A reduced ability of the body to metabolize (use) *glucose,* a form of sugar that is the brain's primary source of fuel. This condition is considered a key feature of *Alzheimer's disease.*

gluten. A mixture of proteins found in wheat, barley, and rye. In people with a form of gluten intolerance, such as *celiac disease,* gluten can cause symptoms ranging from stomach pain to damage of the small intestine.

glycemic index (GI). A system that indicates on a scale of 1 to 100 how quickly a food elevates blood glucose levels. Foods with a high GI cause blood glucose levels to rise quickly. Foods with a low GI increase blood glucose levels more slowly.

glycemic load (GL). A system that indicates the potential of a food to raise blood glucose, based upon the amount of that food eaten and upon the *glycemic index* (GI) of the food. A GL of 20 or more is considered high; one between 11 and 19 is considered medium; and a GL of 10 or less is considered low. Lower GLs are healthier than high GLs.

gut microbiome. The population of *microbes* in the intestines.

high-density lipoprotein (HDL) cholesterol. See *cholesterol.*

high-glycemic food. A food that when eaten causes blood glucose levels to rise relatively quickly. See also *glycemic index.*

hippocampus. The region of the brain that is involved in the formation, organization, storage, and retrieval of memories. The hippocampus is also important in emotional responses, navigation, and spatial orientation.

hyperglycemia. An excess of *glucose* (sugar) in the bloodstream, often associated with *diabetes.*

incomplete protein. A *protein* source (such as wheat) that contains some but not all of the *essential amino acids* that the body needs to function.

insulin. A hormone secreted by the pancreas that allows the body to use *glucose* (a form of sugar metabolized from the carbohydrates in food) to produce energy. If the body has sufficient energy, insulin signals the liver to take up the glucose and store it for future use.

insulin resistance. A condition in which the body's cells have a lower level of response to *insulin,* a hormone secreted by the pancreas to regulate the level of *glucose* (sugar) in the blood by signaling the cells to take in the glucose and convert it to energy. As a result of the cells' resistance, the pancreas produces larger quantities of insulin in an effort to maintain normal blood glucose levels.

intermittent fasting. Also called time-restricted eating, a practice of restricting eating to a small window of time each day.

interval training. A form of exercise, also referred to as speed training or speed work, that alternates bursts of intense activity with periods of lighter activity.

intramuscular fat. Fat stored between the muscles.

ketoacidosis. A life-threatening condition in which high levels of *ketones* cause the blood to become too acidic. Symptoms can include nausea, vomiting, abdominal pain, rapid breathing, and unconsciousness. When this condition is caused by *diabetes*, it is referred to as diabetic ketoacidosis.

ketogenic diet. A diet that promotes the formation of *ketones* through high amounts of fat and significant carbohydrate restriction.

ketones. Organic substances that are created when the body breaks down body fat for fuel, rather than using *glucose* as its fuel source.

ketosis. A metabolic state in which the body burns fragments of fats called *ketones* for fuel instead of burning *glucose.*

legumes. A family of plants that includes beans, peas, and lentils.

low-density lipoprotein (LDL) cholesterol. See *cholesterol.*

low-glycemic food. A food that when eaten causes blood *glucose* levels to rise relatively slowly. See also *glycemic index.*

macronutrients. Nutrients that living organisms need in relatively large amounts to grow, develop, and function. The three major macronutrients are *protein, carbohydrate,* and *fat.*

melatonin. A hormone produced by a gland situated in the brain to regulate sleep-wake cycles. Production of this hormone declines with age, and *Alzheimer's disease* is associated with further decline of melatonin production.

metabolic syndrome. A group of conditions—including high blood pressure, high *blood sugar,* excess body fat around the waist, and abnormal levels of *cholesterol*—that, when they occur together, increase the risk of heart and blood vessel disease, stroke, and diabetes.

microbes. Single-celled microscopic organisms, including bacteria, fungi, protozoa, and viruses.

mild cognitive impairment (MCI). The second stage of *Alzheimer's disease,* commonly characterized by changes in thinking skills that have not yet affected the patient's daily life, but are significant enough to be noticed. Individuals may have recognizable problems with memory, language, or judgment, but these problems do not limit their ability to carry out everyday activities. Mild cognitive impairment can also be described as an intermediate stage between the expected cognitive deterioration associated with aging and the more serious cognitive decline of *dementia.*

mitochondrial dysfunction. Failure of the mitochondria—the specialized components of cells responsible for creating most of the energy needed by the body—to function properly and produce the required amount of energy.

modifiable risk factors. *Risk factors* that can be changed or eliminated, thereby lowering the chance of getting a particular disorder. For example, smoking is a modifiable risk factor for lung cancer, because the individual can stop smoking and thereby reduce the risk of getting cancer.

monounsaturated fats. A type of dietary fat (called "monounsaturated" because each molecule has one unsaturated carbon bond) that is typically liquid at room temperature but begins to turn solid when chilled. Monounsaturated fats can be found in avocados and in many nuts and seeds, including almonds, hazelnuts, pecans, and pumpkin and sesame seeds, as well as in olive, peanut, and canola oils. Because these fats are believed to improve *cholesterol* levels, improve *insulin* levels, and help control *blood sugar,* healthcare professionals generally encourage the consumption of the foods that provide them.

neural pathway. A connection between relatively distant regions of the brain created by nerve axons, the long, slender projections of nerve cells (*neurons*).

neurodegenerative disease. A condition that primarily attacks the *neurons* (brain cells), resulting in a progressive degeneration and/or death of the cells. Neurodegenerative disorders include *Alzheimer's disease,* Parkinson's, and Huntington's disease.

neurons. Also called nerve cells, the specialized cells that carry information to and from the brain via an electrochemical process.

neuroplasticity. Also called brain plasticity, the ability of the brain to form new neural connections and reorganize neural pathways throughout life in response to the individual's experiences. Neuroplasticity can come in two forms: functional plasticity allows the brain to move functions from a damaged area to an undamaged area, and structural plasticity allows it to change its physical structure in response to learning.

neurotransmitters. The chemicals, such as serotonin and acetylcholine, that enable the brain cells to communicate with one another. Neurotransmitters play an important role in regulating body functions such as heartbeat, and also affect mood, concentration, memory, sleep, and more.

NMDA (N-methyl-D-aspartate) antagonists. A category of medications prescribed to manage the symptoms of Alzheimer's disease. NMDA antagonists work by binding to special NMDA receptors for glutamate, and thereby regulating the activity of glutamate, a *neurotransmitter* responsible for memory formation and learning. This category of medications includes Namenda (memantine) and Namzaric (memantine/donepezil).

nonmodifiable risk factors. *Risk factors* that are beyond your control. Age, for instance, constitutes a nonmodifiable risk factor.

nutraceutical. A food or a product derived from food that offers health benefits, including the prevention and/or treatment of disease. It may be a nutrient-rich or medicinally valuable food, such as garlic; or a component of a food, such as omega-3 fatty acids sourced from salmon.

nutrigenomics. Also called nutritional genomics, the study of how foods affect the way the genes grow and behave; how genetic differences can affect the body's response to nutrients and other naturally occurring compounds; and how genes can regulate the body's nutritional requirements.

obesity. A higher-than-healthy weight indicated by a *body mass index* of 30 or more.

omega-3 fatty acids. See *essential fatty acids.*

omega-6 fatty acids. See *essential fatty acids.*

polyunsaturated fats. A type of dietary fat (called "polyunsaturated" because each molecule has more than one unsaturated carbon bond) that is typically liquid at room temperature but begins to turn solid when chilled. Polyunsaturated fats can be found in sunflower, corn, soybean, and flaxseed oils; in some nuts, such as walnuts; and in fatty fish, such as salmon and mackerel. Because these fats are believed to reduce inflammation and lessen the risk of many health problems—including heart disease, stroke, and cancer—healthcare professionals generally encourage the consumption of the foods that provide them. See also *essential fatty acids.*

portion distortion. The phenomenon in which people come to view abnormally large portions of food as being normal. This phenomenon has been attributed to the increased popularity of dining in restaurants, where excessively large portions of food are served to make people feel that they are getting value for their money. The large restaurant portions distort people's image of a normal portion, leading them to prepare and serve excessive portions at home.

prebiotics. Certain nondigestible carbohydrates (fiber) that stimulate the growth of selective gut bacteria.

preclinical Alzheimer's disease. The first stage of *Alzheimer's disease,* in which the individual shows no outwards signs of the disease. In other words, memory and cognitive skills seem to be intact even though the individual's brain has already begun to undergo changes associated with the development of AD.

probiotics. Live bacteria and yeast that promote gut health, and can be ingested in foods such as yogurt as well as in supplements.

protein. One of the *macronutrients,* composed of one or more chains of amino acids. Proteins are fundamental components for all living cells and facilitate many body processes.

pseudobulbar affect (PBA). A condition characterized by uncontrollable, extended outbursts of laughing or crying in people with certain neurological conditions, such as *Alzheimer's disease.*

resistance training. Any exercise that causes muscles to contract against external resistance with the goal of increasing muscle mass, muscle tone, strength, and/or endurance.

risk factors. Traits, characteristics, behaviors, exposures, or conditions that increase the likelihood that a person will develop a certain disorder. See also *modifiable risk factors; nonmodifiable risk factors.*

saturated fat. A type of dietary fat (called "saturated" because it's saturated with hydrogen molecules) that is typically solid at room temperature. Saturated fats are usually of animal origin (examples include butter and the fat found in meat), although they are also found in palm oil, palm kernel oil, and coconut oil. Because a high intake of saturated fat is associated with heart disease and other disorders, healthcare professionals generally advise people to limit their intake of this fat.

selective serotonin reuptake inhibitors (SSRIs). A category of antidepressants. SSRIs work by increasing concentrations in the brain of the *neurotransmitter* serotonin, the so-called happiness hormone. This class of medications includes Celexa (citalopram), Lexapro (escitalopram), and Cipralex (escitalopram).

simple carbohydrates. See *carbohydrates.*

speed training. See *interval training.*

structural plasticity. See *neuroplasticity.*

subcutaneous fat. Excess fat stored under the skin.

synergy. The interaction of two or more substances or strategies that produces a combined effect which is greater than the sum of the separate benefits.

tau tangles. Twisted protein threads composed of a protein called tau that form within nerve cells (*neurons*), preventing them from communicating with one another and eventually leading to nerve cell death. Also called neurofibrillary tangles, they are considered one of the hallmarks of *Alzheimer's disease.*

time-restricted eating. See *intermittent fasting.*

trans fats. A type of dietary fat—some of which is naturally occurring and some of which is artificially produced—that is believed to increase "bad" LDL cholesterol and decrease "good" HDL cholesterol. Naturally occurring trans fats are found in only small quantities in some meat and dairy products. The primary dietary source of this harmful fat is partially hydrogenated oils, which are created industrially and used to make many prepared foods, including doughnuts, many types of baked goods, stick margarines, and frozen pizzas. Because it is considered the most damaging type of fat, many health-care professionals advise the total elimination of trans fats from the diet. These fats are also referred to as trans fatty acids.

type 1 diabetes. See *diabetes.*

type 2 diabetes. See *diabetes.*

vascular dementia. The second most common form of *dementia,* caused by impaired blood supply to the brain. This disorder can be the result of stroke or of other conditions that damage blood vessels or reduce circulation, depriving the brain of nutrients and oxygen.

visceral fat. Fat stored in and around the internal organs, such as the stomach and liver. This form of fat has been identified as posing a danger to the body because it pumps out harmful chemicals that can lead to negative health consequences such as heart disease, high cholesterol, and insulin resistance.

younger-onset Alzheimer's disease. See *early-onset Alzheimer's disease.*

Resources

A number of organizations and websites provide a wealth of information on Alzheimer's disease, its risk factors, its stages, its management, and other topics of interest to the person who seeks to prevent or slow Alzheimer's disease or has a family member with AD. Below, you'll find a listing of those organizations that particularly focus on AD, as well as websites that will help you find the nutritional information you need to choose your foods wisely; calculate and understand BMI and other aspects of health; and maintain or improve cognitive function. Finally, you'll find organizations geared to assist families that serve as caregivers for loved ones with AD, and websites that provide information about nutritional supplements and AD. Note that although we have organized the resources into handy categories, some of these resources provide multiple services—such as general AD information *plus* caregiver support—so it makes sense to visit the various websites and see what each has to offer.

GENERAL ALZHEIMER'S INFORMATION AND SUPPORT

Alzheimer's Association (AA)
225 North Michigan Avenue, Floor 17
Chicago, IL 60601
Phone: (312) 335-8700
Helpline: (800) 272-3900
Website: www.alz.org

The Alzheimer's Association is a leading voluntary health organization in AD care, support, education, and research. Visit its website to find extensive information on the disease; local support groups; a guide to community Alzheimer's programs and events, housing options, and other care options; help with financial and legal matters; information on clinical trials; and more. A twenty-four-hour helpline is also available.

Alzheimer's Disease Education and Referral Center (ADEAR)

National Institute on Aging
Building 31, Room 5C27
31 Center Drive, MSC 2292
Bethesda, MD 20892
Phone: (800) 438-4380
Website: www.nia.nih.gov/alzheimers

Part of the National Institute on Aging, the Alzheimer's Disease Education and Referral Center teaches users about AD and offers extensive information on Alzheimer's initiatives, current trials, and support. A variety of fact sheets and other publications are available online.

Alzheimer's Foundation of American (AFA)

322 Eighth Avenue, 7th Floor
New York, NY 10001
Phone: (646) 638-1542
Toll-free Helpline: (866) 232-8484
Website: www.alzfdn.org

With the primary mission of ensuring good care for people with Alzheimer's disease and their families, the AFA offers educational resources and support. Its toll-free helpline—available Monday through Friday and staffed by licensed social workers—provides direction and assistance to individual care providers and families who are coping with AD.

AlzRisk AD Epidemiology Database

1 Main Street, 13th Floor
Cambridge, MA 02142
Website: www.AlzRisk.org

Run by AlzForum, a clearinghouse for AD research, the AlzRisk AD Epidemiology Database collects information on nongenetic AD risk factors, summarizing and evaluating current studies to help you understand how different environmental factors contribute to the likelihood of developing AD.

National Institute of Neurological Disorders and Stroke

NIH Neurological Institute

P.O. Box 5801

Bethesda, MD 20824

Phone: (800) 352-9424

Website: http://www.ninds.nih.gov/disorders/alzheimersdisease/
alzheimersdisease.htm

The mission of this institute is to seek fundamental knowledge about the brain and nervous system and to use that knowledge to reduce the burden of neurological disease. In addition to offering basic information on Alzheimer's disease, the website provides links to a variety of helpful organizations, including those that offer support for caregivers and help families locate respite care.

NUTRITIONAL DATA

Harvard Health Publications—Glycemic Index and Glycemic Load

Website: http://www.health.harvard.edu/healthy-eating/
glycemic_index_and_glycemic_load_for_100_foods

This publication of Harvard Medical School provides the glycemic index and glycemic load of more than one hundred foods, which are broken into categories such as Bakery Products and Breads, Beverages, Breakfast Cereals, Cookies and Crackers, etc. Although more limited in size than the Mendosa.com list, this guide makes it easier to find generic foods such as brown rice, as well as some popular brand-name products.

Mendosa.com

David Mendosa

993 E. Moorhead, Circle Suite 2F

Boulder, CO 80305

Phone: (720) 319-8423

Website: http://www.mendosa.com/gilists.htm

Developed by medical writer David Mendosa to help people with diabetes, Mendosa.com is the authors' favorite website for finding the glycemic index (GI) and glycemic load (GL) of foods. The listing provides the GI and GL of more than 2,480 individual food items. Be aware, though, that the list, although long, includes foods from many different countries. In other words, many of the products are not available in the United States.

Self Nutrition Data

Website: www.nutritiondata.com

This website provides complete nutritional data—including carbohydrate counts—for individual foods, both plain and prepared. Just plug the name of the food into the search feature.

Supertracker

USDA Center for Nutrition Policy and Promotion
3101 Park Center Drive, Room 1034
Alexandria, VA 22302
Phone: (888) 779-7264
Website: https://supertracker.usda.gov/

Created by the United States Department of Agriculture, SuperTracker makes it easy to get detailed nutritional information and track your diet. Click on the "Food-A-Pedia" tab, and you'll be able to access full nutritional data—calories, protein, carbohydrates, fiber, sugars, saturated fat, and more—for a wide range of fresh foods and brand-name products. The site also helps you build a list of favorite foods, and links foods together to evaluate a recipe that has multiple ingredients.

USDA National Nutrient Database for Standard Reference

Website: http://ndb.nal.usda.gov/

Created by the United States Department of Agriculture, this database provides nutrition information—including carbohydrate counts—for nearly 9,000 foods. Enter the item in the search feature or look through an alphabetical list to find a complete analysis of nutrients.

MAINTAINING AND IMPROVING COGNITIVE FUNCTION

Alzheimer's Universe

General Website: www.AlzU.org
Nutrition Tracking System Website:
  http://www.alzheimersdiet.com/alzu/

Created by Weill Cornell Medicine and NewYork-Presbyterian and collaborators from throughout the world, this site provides a variety of lessons and activities to help you optimize and understand a comprehensive approach to brain health. You will begin by completing a five- to ten-minute questionnaire, followed by lessons and activities. The more lessons you complete, the more lessons will "unlock," and the more you will learn about overall brain health. Alzheimer's Universe also provides a Nutrition Tracking System (AD-NTS) that will allow you to track your progress as you follow the Alzheimer's Prevention and Treatment Diet.

Therapy for Memory

Phone: 786-4-MEMORY

Website: http://www.therapyformemory.org/

This website is dedicated to providing up-to-date information and resources for people with AD and their caregivers, family, and healthcare providers. Information is presented on using different strategies to fight memory loss, including education, diet, vitamins, music, physical exercise, and mental exercise. Features include an "Ask the Experts" section, where you can submit questions to the site's resident clinicians.

CALCULATING BMI AND OTHER RISK FACTORS

Centers for Disease Control and Prevention—BMI Calculator

1600 Clifton Road

Atlanta, GA 30329-4027

Phone: 800-232-4636

Website: http://www.cdc.gov/healthyweight/assessing/bmi/

The CDC provides information on body mass index (BMI), as well as a BMI calculator and information on interpreting the BMI for both adults and younger people.

Global Vascular Risk Score Calculator

Website: http://neurology.med.miami.edu/gvr

This site of the University of Miami Miller School of Medicine allows you to calculate your GVRS, or Global Vascular Risk Score, by typing in information such as age, ethnicity, systolic blood pressure, and diastolic blood pressure. Because vascular damage is a major risk factor for brain shrinkage and cognitive decline, the GVRS can be a useful tool in helping determine and modify cardiovascular risk that may adversely affect the brain.

National Heart, Lung, and Blood Institute (NHLBI)

P.O. Box 30105

Bethesda, MD 20824

Phone: 301-592-8573

Website: http://www.nhlbi.nih.gov/health/educational/lose_wt/BMI/ bmicalc.htm

To help you assess your weight and health risk, the NHLBI provides a BMI calculator, information on waist circumference, and information on health issues associated with obesity.

FINDING CAREGIVER SUPPORT PROGRAMS AND AGENCIES

Family Caregiver Alliance (FCA)

785 Market Street, Suite 750
San Francisco, CA 94103
Phone: (800) 445-8106
Website: www.caregiver.org

The FCA was the first community-based nonprofit organization in the United States to address the needs of those who provide long-term care for loved ones at home. Among the services offered on its website is a Family Care Navigator—a state-by-state guide to help families locate government, nonprofit, and private caregiver support programs. The Navigator lists programs for family caregivers as well as resources for older or disabled adults living at home or in a residential facility. Fact sheets and publications on a variety of caregiving topics and health issues are available.

Medicare.gov Home Health Compare

Website: www.medicare.gov / HomeHealthCompare /

Part of the official United States Government site for Medicare, this feature uses a "quality of patient care star rating" to show how the performance of a given Medicare-certified home health agency compares with that of other Medicare-certified agencies. The star rating summarizes the agency's average performance on measured care practices, including managing daily activities, managing pain and treating symptoms, treating wounds and preventing bed sores, preventing harm, and avoiding unplanned hospital care.

NUTRITIONAL SUPPLEMENTS

Alzheimer's Drug Discovery Foundation—Cognitive Vitality

57 West 57th Street, Suite 904
New York, NY 10019
Phone: (212) 901-8000
Website: www.alzdiscovery.org / cognitive-vitality

Founded in 1998, this foundation provides funding to leading scientists who are conducting Alzheimer's drug research worldwide. It also evaluates strategies that have been proposed to prevent brain aging, Alzheimer's disease, and related dementias. A special section reviews supplements, traditional herbs, nutraceuticals, and other natural products, examining each substance's ability to protect the brain and prevent cognitive decline.

Carlson Laboratories

600 West University Drive
Arlington Heights, IL 60004
Phone: (800) 323-4141
Website: www.carlsonlabs.com

Carlson Laboratories produces high-quality nutritional supplements, including fish oil soft gels, which provide omega-3s EPA and DHA sourced from deep cold-water fish using sustainable methods. Carlson's fish oils are tested by an FDA-registered laboratory for freshness, potency, and purity.

CocoaVia

Phone: (877) 842-0802
Website: www.cocoavia.com

CocoaVia supplements provide guaranteed amounts of cocoa flavanols. The supplements are available as capsules and as dark chocolate stick packs, which contain a powder that can be stirred into beverages and yogurt.

National Center for Complementary and Integrative Health (NCCIH)

US Department of Health and Human Services
9000 Rockville Pike
Bethesda, MD 20892
Phone: (888-644-6226
Website: https://nccih.nih.gov/health/providers/digest/alzheimers-science

The NCCIH is the Federal Government's lead agency for scientific research on the medical and health care systems, practices, and products that are generally not considered part of conventional medicine. Its online article on dietary supplements and cognitive function, dementia, and Alzheimer's looks at several supplements that have been studied for their potential to prevent or treat Alzheimer's disease.

Nutrition
and Activity Logs

In Chapter 5, which presents the Alzheimer's Prevention and Treatment Diet, we encourage you to record certain aspects of your diet and lifestyle. We also ask you to record your favorite foods and meals. Keeping track of your diet and other brain-healthy activities has been shown to be extremely valuable, regardless of the food plan you're following. It instantly increases your awareness of what, how much, and why you are eating. It also helps you identify the areas in which you may need to make changes. For instance, when you record the carbohydrate counts of the foods you eat, you'll become more aware of foods that provide a high amount of carbohydrates, and therefore may have to be limited on (or eliminated from) your diet. (See page 231 of the Resources list for websites that list carb counts for various foods. When using packaged foods, check the Nutrition Facts label.) Because we also ask you to compile lists of the snacks, foods, and meals that you prefer, you will always have a reference you can turn to when you need a menu idea.

Many people like to keep a paper record, such as the one we provide below. But if you prefer to record your progress on the computer, log onto the Nutrition Tracking System (AD-NTS) found on the Alzheimer's Universe website. (See page 232 of the Resources list for contact information.)

WEEK 1 OF THE APT DIET

In Week 1 of the APT Diet, you will not be making any changes to your usual diet and lifestyle activities, but will be "taking stock" by noting some of the *unhealthy* snacks and foods that you customarily eat—and that you will have to limit or eliminate on your new diet—and by totaling carb consumption for two days. You will also prepare for Week 2 by coming up with some exercises that you can perform in the coming weeks. Finally, you will record your weight to set your baseline.

■ **Record three favorite brain-*un*healthy snacks (which you will eventually replace).**

1._____

2._____

3._____

■ **Record three favorite brain-*un*healthy meals (which you will eventually replace).**

1._____

2._____

3._____

■ **Write down five of the brain-unhealthy foods you have in your pantry and refrigerator, and come up with solutions to these diet challenges—such as buying them in limited quantities, replacing them with healthier foods, or simply eliminating them from your kitchen.**

1. Unhealthy food_____

   Solution _____

2. Unhealthy food_____

   Solution _____

3. Unhealthy food_____

   Solution _____

4. Unhealthy food_____

   Solution _____

5. Unhealthy food_____

   Solution _____

■ **For two days—one weekday and one weekend day—write down everything you eat, and note the total grams of carbohydrates found in the portion you consumed. Then total your carb grams for that day. This will make you aware of the amount of carbohydrates you usually consume.**

DAY 1

Food _____ Carb grams _____

Food _____ Carb grams _____

Food _____ Carb grams _____

Food _____ Carb grams _____

Food _____ Carb grams _____

Food _____ Carb grams _____

Food _____ Carb grams _____

Food _____ Carb grams _____

Food _____ Carb grams _____

Food _____ Carb grams _____

Food _____ Carb grams _____

Food _____ Carb grams _____

                                        Total carbs _____

Day 2

Food _____ Carb grams _____

Food _____ Carb grams _____

Food _____ Carb grams _____

Food _____ Carb grams _____

Food _____ Carb grams _____

Food _____ Carb grams _____

Food _____ Carb grams _____

Food _____ Carb grams _____

Food _____ Carb grams _____

Food _____ Carb grams _____

Food _____ Carb grams _____

Food _____ Carb grams _____

Food _____ Carb grams _____

Total carbs _____

■ **Identify and write down several exercises that you could perform for at least 20 minutes at a time, three times each week.**

Exercise 1 _____

Exercise 2 _____

Exercise 3 _____

Exercise 4 _____

Exercise 5 _____

■ **Record your weight to set your baseline:** _____

WEEK 2 OF THE APT DIET

In Week 2, you will begin following the APT Diet (as detailed on page 122) and implementing lifestyle changes. Below, you can keep track of your carbohydrate consumption to make sure that you're following the Week 2 guidelines. You can also record your exercise sessions, any brain-engaging activities you choose, and any stress-reducing activities you decide to try. If you come up with new ideas for brain-healthy meals and snacks, we encourage you to write them in your log (see the end of the Week 2 log) so that you will be able to refer to your notes whenever you need some good menu ideas.

■ **Each day of Week 2, write down the foods you eat along with their carbohydrate counts. This will allow you to track your carbs throughout the day so that you can stick to your Week 2 limit of 140 to 160 grams. At the end of each day, record your carb total.**

SUNDAY

Food _____ Carb grams _____

Food _____ Carb grams _____

Food _____ Carb grams _____

Food _____ Carb grams _____

Food _____ Carb grams _____

Food _____ Carb grams _____

Food _____ Carb grams _____

Food _____ Carb grams _____

Food _____ Carb grams _____

Food _____ Carb grams _____

Total carbs _____

MONDAY

Food _____ Carb grams _____

Food _____ Carb grams _____

Food _____ Carb grams _____

Food _____ Carb grams _____

Food _____ Carb grams _____

Food _____ Carb grams _____

Food _____ Carb grams _____

Food _____ Carb grams _____

Food _____ Carb grams _____

Food _____ Carb grams _____

Total carbs _____

TUESDAY

Food _____ Carb grams _____

Food _____ Carb grams _____

Food _____ Carb grams _____

Food _____ Carb grams _____

Food _____ Carb grams _____

Food _____ Carb grams _____

Food _____ Carb grams _____

Food _____ Carb grams _____

Food _____ Carb grams _____

Food _____ Carb grams _____

Total carbs _____

WEDNESDAY

Food _____ Carb grams _____

Food _____ Carb grams _____

Food _____ Carb grams _____

Food _____ Carb grams _____

Food _____ Carb grams _____

Food _____ Carb grams _____

Food _____ Carb grams _____

Food _____ Carb grams _____

Food _____ Carb grams _____

Food _____ Carb grams _____

Total carbs _____

THURSDAY

Food _____ Carb grams _____

Food _____ Carb grams _____

Food _____ Carb grams _____

Food _____ Carb grams _____

Food _____ Carb grams _____

Food _____ Carb grams _____

Food _____ Carb grams _____

Food _____ Carb grams _____

Food _____ Carb grams _____

Food _____ Carb grams _____

Total carbs _____

FRIDAY

Food _____ Carb grams _____

Food _____ Carb grams _____

Food _____ Carb grams _____

Food _____ Carb grams _____

Food _____ Carb grams _____

Food _____ Carb grams _____

Food _____ Carb grams _____

Food _____ Carb grams _____

Food _____ Carb grams _____

Food _____ Carb grams _____

Total carbs _____

SATURDAY

Food _____ Carb grams _____

Food _____ Carb grams _____

Food _____ Carb grams _____

Food _____ Carb grams _____

Food _____ Carb grams _____

Food _____ Carb grams _____

Food _____ Carb grams _____

Food _____ Carb grams _____

Food _____ Carb grams _____

Food _____ Carb grams _____

Total carbs _____

■ **Record your exercise sessions for Week 2.**

Exercise _____ Duration _____minutes

Exercise _____ Duration _____minutes

■ **Record your brain-engaging activities for Week 2.**

_____

_____

_____

_____

_____

■ **Record your stress-reducing activities for Week 2.**

_____

_____

_____

_____

■ **Record new ideas for brain-healthy meals and/or snacks that you plan to prepare or have already prepared.**

Breakfast _____

_____

Lunch _____

_____

Dinner _____

_____

Snacks _____

_____

WEEK 3 OF THE APT DIET

In Week 3, you will continue adjusting your diet to make it more brain-healthy (as detailed on page 128) and will also track your carbs, just as you did during Week 2. For the best results, make note of your exercise sessions, brain-engaging activities, and stress-reducing activities, as well as any new ideas you have for snacks and meals.

■ **Each day of Week 3, write down the foods you eat along with their carbohydrate counts. This will allow you to track your carbs throughout the day so that you can stick to your Week 3 limit of 140 to 160 grams. At the end of each day, record your carb total.**

SUNDAY

Food _____ Carb grams _____

Food _____ Carb grams _____

Food _____ Carb grams _____

Food _____ Carb grams _____

Food _____ Carb grams _____

Food _____ Carb grams _____

Food _____ Carb grams _____

Food _____ Carb grams _____

Food _____ Carb grams _____

Food _____ Carb grams _____

Food _____ Carb grams _____

Food _____ Carb grams _____

Food _____ Carb grams _____

Total carbs _____

MONDAY

Food _____   Carb grams _____

Food _____   Carb grams _____

Food _____   Carb grams _____

Food _____   Carb grams _____

Food _____   Carb grams _____

Food _____   Carb grams _____

Food _____   Carb grams _____

Food _____   Carb grams _____

Food _____   Carb grams _____

Food _____   Carb grams _____

                                        Total carbs _____

TUESDAY

Food _____   Carb grams _____

Food _____   Carb grams _____

Food _____   Carb grams _____

Food _____   Carb grams _____

Food _____   Carb grams _____

Food _____   Carb grams _____

Food _____   Carb grams _____

Food _____   Carb grams _____

Food _____   Carb grams _____

Food _____   Carb grams _____

                                        Total carbs _____

WEDNESDAY

Food _____ Carb grams _____

Food _____ Carb grams _____

Food _____ Carb grams _____

Food _____ Carb grams _____

Food _____ Carb grams _____

Food _____ Carb grams _____

Food _____ Carb grams _____

Food _____ Carb grams _____

Food _____ Carb grams _____

Food _____ Carb grams _____

Total carbs _____

THURSDAY

Food _____ Carb grams _____

Food _____ Carb grams _____

Food _____ Carb grams _____

Food _____ Carb grams _____

Food _____ Carb grams _____

Food _____ Carb grams _____

Food _____ Carb grams _____

Food _____ Carb grams _____

Food _____ Carb grams _____

Food _____ Carb grams _____

Total carbs _____

FRIDAY

Food _____ Carb grams _____

Food _____ Carb grams _____

Food _____ Carb grams _____

Food _____ Carb grams _____

Food _____ Carb grams _____

Food _____ Carb grams _____

Food _____ Carb grams _____

Food _____ Carb grams _____

Food _____ Carb grams _____

Food _____ Carb grams _____

Total carbs _____

SATURDAY

Food _____ Carb grams _____

Food _____ Carb grams _____

Food _____ Carb grams _____

Food _____ Carb grams _____

Food _____ Carb grams _____

Food _____ Carb grams _____

Food _____ Carb grams _____

Food _____ Carb grams _____

Food _____ Carb grams _____

Food _____ Carb grams _____

Total carbs _____

■ **Record your exercise sessions for Week 3.**

Exercise _____ Duration _____minutes

Exercise _____ Duration _____minutes

Exercise _____ Duration _____minutes

Exercise _____ Duration _____minutes

■ **Record your brain-engaging activities for Week 3.**

_____

_____

_____

_____

_____

■ **Record your stress-reducing activities for Week 3.**

_____

_____

_____

_____

_____

■ **Record new ideas for brain-healthy meals and/or snacks that you plan to prepare or have already prepared.**

Breakfast _____

Lunch _____

Dinner _____

Snacks _____

WEEK 4 OF THE APT DIET

In Week 4, you will continue adjusting your diet to make it more brain-healthy (as detailed on page 131) and will also track your carbs, just as you did during Week 3. For the best results, note your exercise sessions, brain-engaging activities, and stress-reducing activities, as well as any new ideas you have for snacks and meals. Because you want to be able to comfortably follow the APT Diet even when you're away from home, take a little time to come up with ideas for "portable" foods you can prepare in advance or buy at a restaurant. Note that at the end of this week, you should record your weight again, ideally using the same scale you used when you began following the diet.

■ **Record two brain-healthy meals (aside from meal replacements) that can be consumed outside the home for breakfast, lunch, and dinner. These meals can be prepared in advance and taken with you, or purchased from a restaurant or market.**

Breakfast _____

_____

Lunch _____

_____

Dinner _____

_____

Snacks _____

_____

■ **Each day of Week 4, write down the foods you eat along with their carbohydrate counts. This will allow you to track your carbs throughout the day so that you can to stick to your Week 4 limit of 130 to 140 grams. At the end of each day, record your carb total.**

SUNDAY

Food _____   Carb grams _____

Food _____   Carb grams _____

Food _____   Carb grams _____

Food _____   Carb grams _____

Food _____   Carb grams _____

Food _____   Carb grams _____

Food _____   Carb grams _____

Food _____   Carb grams _____

Food _____   Carb grams _____

Food _____   Carb grams _____

Total carbs _____

MONDAY

Food _____   Carb grams _____

Food _____   Carb grams _____

Food _____   Carb grams _____

Food _____   Carb grams _____

Food _____   Carb grams _____

Food _____   Carb grams _____

Food _____   Carb grams _____

Food _____   Carb grams _____

Food _____   Carb grams _____

Food _____   Carb grams _____

Total carbs _____

TUESDAY

Food _____ Carb grams _____

Food _____ Carb grams _____

Food _____ Carb grams _____

Food _____ Carb grams _____

Food _____ Carb grams _____

Food _____ Carb grams _____

Food _____ Carb grams _____

Food _____ Carb grams _____

Food _____ Carb grams _____

Food _____ Carb grams _____

Total carbs _____

WEDNESDAY

Food _____ Carb grams _____

Food _____ Carb grams _____

Food _____ Carb grams _____

Food _____ Carb grams _____

Food _____ Carb grams _____

Food _____ Carb grams _____

Food _____ Carb grams _____

Food _____ Carb grams _____

Food _____ Carb grams _____

Food _____ Carb grams _____

Total carbs _____

THURSDAY

Food _____ Carb grams _____

Food _____ Carb grams _____

Food _____ Carb grams _____

Food _____ Carb grams _____

Food _____ Carb grams _____

Food _____ Carb grams _____

Food _____ Carb grams _____

Food _____ Carb grams _____

Food _____ Carb grams _____

Food _____ Carb grams _____

Total carbs _____

FRIDAY

Food _____ Carb grams _____

Food _____ Carb grams _____

Food _____ Carb grams _____

Food _____ Carb grams _____

Food _____ Carb grams _____

Food _____ Carb grams _____

Food _____ Carb grams _____

Food _____ Carb grams _____

Food _____ Carb grams _____

Food _____ Carb grams _____

Total carbs _____

SATURDAY

Food _____ Carb grams _____

Food _____ Carb grams _____

Food _____ Carb grams _____

Food _____ Carb grams _____

Food _____ Carb grams _____

Food _____ Carb grams _____

Food _____ Carb grams _____

Food _____ Carb grams _____

Food _____ Carb grams _____

Food _____ Carb grams _____

Food _____ Carb grams _____

Food _____ Carb grams _____

Food _____ Carb grams _____

Food _____ Carb grams _____

Total carbs _____

■ **Record your exercise sessions for Week 4.**

Exercise _____ Duration _____minutes

Exercise _____ Duration _____minutes

Exercise _____ Duration _____minutes

Exercise _____ Duration _____minutes

Exercise _____ Duration _____minutes

Exercise _____ Duration _____minutes

■ Record your brain-engaging activities for Week 4.

_____

_____

_____

_____

_____

_____

■ Record your stress-reducing activities for Week 4.

_____

_____

_____

_____

_____

■ Record new ideas for brain-healthy meals and/or snacks that you plan to prepare or have already prepared.

Breakfast _____

_____

Lunch _____

_____

Dinner _____

_____

Snacks _____

_____

■ Record your weight at Week 4: _____

WEEK 5 OF THE APT DIET

In Week 5, you will continue adjusting your diet to make it more brain-healthy (as detailed on page 135) and will also track your carbohydrates, just as you did during Week 4. For the best results, note your exercise sessions, brain-engaging activities, and stress-reducing activities, as well as any new ideas you have for snacks and meals.

■ **Identify and record three challenges to eating outside the home, and two potential solutions to each challenge.**

Challenge to eating out _____

Possible solution _____

_____

_____

Possible solution _____

_____

_____

Challenge to eating out _____

Possible solution _____

_____

_____

Possible solution _____

_____

_____

■ **Each day of Week 5, write down the foods you eat along with their carbohydrate counts. This will allow you to track your carbs throughout the day so that you can stick to your Week 5 limit of 130 to 140 grams. At the end of each day, record your carb total.**

SUNDAY

Food _____ Carb grams _____

Food _____ Carb grams _____

Food _____ Carb grams _____

Food _____ Carb grams _____

Food _____ Carb grams _____

Food _____ Carb grams _____

Food _____ Carb grams _____

Food _____ Carb grams _____

Food _____ Carb grams _____

Food _____ Carb grams _____

Total carbs _____

MONDAY

Food _____ Carb grams _____

Food _____ Carb grams _____

Food _____ Carb grams _____

Food _____ Carb grams _____

Food _____ Carb grams _____

Food _____ Carb grams _____

Food _____ Carb grams _____

Food _____ Carb grams _____

Food _____ Carb grams _____

Food _____ Carb grams _____

Total carbs _____

TUESDAY

Food _____ Carb grams _____

Food _____ Carb grams _____

Food _____ Carb grams _____

Food _____ Carb grams _____

Food _____ Carb grams _____

Food _____ Carb grams _____

Food _____ Carb grams _____

Food _____ Carb grams _____

Food _____ Carb grams _____

Food _____ Carb grams _____

Total carbs _____

WEDNESDAY

Food _____ Carb grams _____

Food _____ Carb grams _____

Food _____ Carb grams _____

Food _____ Carb grams _____

Food _____ Carb grams _____

Food _____ Carb grams _____

Food _____ Carb grams _____

Food _____ Carb grams _____

Food _____ Carb grams _____

Food _____ Carb grams _____

Total carbs _____

THURSDAY

Food _____ Carb grams _____

Food _____ Carb grams _____

Food _____ Carb grams _____

Food _____ Carb grams _____

Food _____ Carb grams _____

Food _____ Carb grams _____

Food _____ Carb grams _____

Food _____ Carb grams _____

Food _____ Carb grams _____

Food _____ Carb grams _____

Total carbs _____

FRIDAY

Food _____ Carb grams _____

Food _____ Carb grams _____

Food _____ Carb grams _____

Food _____ Carb grams _____

Food _____ Carb grams _____

Food _____ Carb grams _____

Food _____ Carb grams _____

Food _____ Carb grams _____

Food _____ Carb grams _____

Food _____ Carb grams _____

Total carbs _____

SATURDAY

Food _____ Carb grams _____

Food _____ Carb grams _____

Food _____ Carb grams _____

Food _____ Carb grams _____

Food _____ Carb grams _____

Food _____ Carb grams _____

Food _____ Carb grams _____

Food _____ Carb grams _____

Food _____ Carb grams _____

Food _____ Carb grams _____

Total carbs _____

■ **Record your exercise sessions for Week 5.**

Exercise _____ Duration _____minutes

Exercise _____ Duration _____minutes

Exercise _____ Duration _____minutes

Exercise _____ Duration _____minutes

Exercise _____ Duration _____minutes

■ **Record your brain-engaging activities for Week 5.**

_____

_____

_____

_____

_____

■ **Record your stress-reducing activities for Week 5.**

_____

_____

_____

_____

_____

_____

_____

_____

■ **Record new ideas for brain-healthy meals and/or snacks that you plan to prepare or have already prepared.**

Breakfast _____

_____

_____

Lunch _____

_____

_____

Dinner _____

_____

_____

Snacks _____

_____

_____

WEEK 6 OF THE APT DIET

In Week 6, you will continue adjusting your diet to make it more brain-healthy (as detailed on page 138) and will also track your carbohydrates, just as you did during Week 5. For the best results, note your exercise sessions, brain-engaging activities, and stress-reducing activities, as well as any new ideas you have for snacks and meals.

■ **Each day of Week 6, write down the foods you eat along with their carbohydrate counts. This will allow you to track your carbs throughout the day so that you can stick to your Week 6 limit of 120 to 130 grams. At the end of each day, record your carb total.**

SUNDAY

Food _____ Carb grams _____

Food _____ Carb grams _____

Food _____ Carb grams _____

Food _____ Carb grams _____

Food _____ Carb grams _____

Food _____ Carb grams _____

Food _____ Carb grams _____

Food _____ Carb grams _____

Food _____ Carb grams _____

Food _____ Carb grams _____

Food _____ Carb grams _____

Food _____ Carb grams _____

Total carbs _____

MONDAY

Food _____ Carb grams _____

Food _____ Carb grams _____

Food _____ Carb grams _____

Food _____ Carb grams _____

Food _____ Carb grams _____

Food _____ Carb grams _____

Food _____ Carb grams _____

Food _____ Carb grams _____

Food _____ Carb grams _____

Food _____ Carb grams _____

Total carbs _____

TUESDAY

Food _____ Carb grams _____

Food _____ Carb grams _____

Food _____ Carb grams _____

Food _____ Carb grams _____

Food _____ Carb grams _____

Food _____ Carb grams _____

Food _____ Carb grams _____

Food _____ Carb grams _____

Food _____ Carb grams _____

Food _____ Carb grams _____

Total carbs _____

WEDNESDAY

Food _____ Carb grams _____

Food _____ Carb grams _____

Food _____ Carb grams _____

Food _____ Carb grams _____

Food _____ Carb grams _____

Food _____ Carb grams _____

Food _____ Carb grams _____

Food _____ Carb grams _____

Food _____ Carb grams _____

Food _____ Carb grams _____

Total carbs _____

THURSDAY

Food _____ Carb grams _____

Food _____ Carb grams _____

Food _____ Carb grams _____

Food _____ Carb grams _____

Food _____ Carb grams _____

Food _____ Carb grams _____

Food _____ Carb grams _____

Food _____ Carb grams _____

Food _____ Carb grams _____

Food _____ Carb grams _____

Total carbs _____

FRIDAY

Food _____ Carb grams _____

Food _____ Carb grams _____

Food _____ Carb grams _____

Food _____ Carb grams _____

Food _____ Carb grams _____

Food _____ Carb grams _____

Food _____ Carb grams _____

Food _____ Carb grams _____

Food _____ Carb grams _____

Food _____ Carb grams _____

Total carbs _____

SATURDAY

Food _____ Carb grams _____

Food _____ Carb grams _____

Food _____ Carb grams _____

Food _____ Carb grams _____

Food _____ Carb grams _____

Food _____ Carb grams _____

Food _____ Carb grams _____

Food _____ Carb grams _____

Food _____ Carb grams _____

Food _____ Carb grams _____

Total carbs _____

■ **Record your exercise sessions for Week 6.**

Exercise _____ Duration _____minutes

Exercise _____ Duration _____minutes

Exercise _____ Duration _____minutes

Exercise _____ Duration _____minutes

Exercise _____ Duration _____minutes

■ **Record your brain-engaging activities for Week 6.**

_____

_____

_____

_____

_____

■ **Record your stress-reducing activities for Week 6.**

_____

_____

_____

_____

_____

■ **Record new ideas for brain-healthy meals and/or snacks that you plan to prepare or have already prepared.**

Breakfast _____

Lunch _____

Dinner _____

Snacks _____

WEEK 7 OF THE APT DIET

In Week 7, you will continue adjusting your diet to make it more brain-healthy (as detailed on page 141) and will also track your carbs, just as you did during Week 6. For the best results, note your exercise sessions, brain-engaging activities, and stress-reducing activities, as well as any new ideas you have for snacks and meals. At the end of this week, you should record your weight again, ideally using the same scale you used when you began the diet and in Week 4.

■ **Each day of Week 7, write down the foods you eat along with their carbohydrate counts. This will allow you to track your carbs throughout the day so that you can to stick to your Week 4 limit of 120 to 130 grams. At the end of each day, record your carb total.**

SUNDAY

Food _____ Carb grams _____

Food _____ Carb grams _____

Food _____ Carb grams _____

Food _____ Carb grams _____

Food _____ Carb grams _____

Food _____ Carb grams _____

Food _____ Carb grams _____

Food _____ Carb grams _____

Food _____ Carb grams _____

Food _____ Carb grams _____

Food _____ Carb grams _____

Total carbs _____

MONDAY

Food _____ Carb grams _____

Food _____ Carb grams _____

Food _____ Carb grams _____

Food _____ Carb grams _____

Food _____ Carb grams _____

Food _____ Carb grams _____

Food _____ Carb grams _____

Food _____ Carb grams _____

Food _____ Carb grams _____

Food _____ Carb grams _____

Total carbs _____

TUESDAY

Food _____ Carb grams _____

Food _____ Carb grams _____

Food _____ Carb grams _____

Food _____ Carb grams _____

Food _____ Carb grams _____

Food _____ Carb grams _____

Food _____ Carb grams _____

Food _____ Carb grams _____

Food _____ Carb grams _____

Food _____ Carb grams _____

Total carbs _____

WEDNESDAY

Food _____ Carb grams _____

Food _____ Carb grams _____

Food _____ Carb grams _____

Food _____ Carb grams _____

Food _____ Carb grams _____

Food _____ Carb grams _____

Food _____ Carb grams _____

Food _____ Carb grams _____

Food _____ Carb grams _____

Food _____ Carb grams _____

Total carbs _____

THURSDAY

Food _____ Carb grams _____

Food _____ Carb grams _____

Food _____ Carb grams _____

Food _____ Carb grams _____

Food _____ Carb grams _____

Food _____ Carb grams _____

Food _____ Carb grams _____

Food _____ Carb grams _____

Food _____ Carb grams _____

Food _____ Carb grams _____

Total carbs _____

FRIDAY

Food _____ Carb grams _____

Food _____ Carb grams _____

Food _____ Carb grams _____

Food _____ Carb grams _____

Food _____ Carb grams _____

Food _____ Carb grams _____

Food _____ Carb grams _____

Food _____ Carb grams _____

Food _____ Carb grams _____

Food _____ Carb grams _____

Total carbs _____

SATURDAY

Food _____ Carb grams _____

Food _____ Carb grams _____

Food _____ Carb grams _____

Food _____ Carb grams _____

Food _____ Carb grams _____

Food _____ Carb grams _____

Food _____ Carb grams _____

Food _____ Carb grams _____

Food _____ Carb grams _____

Food _____ Carb grams _____

Total carbs _____

■ **Record your exercise sessions for Week 7.**

Exercise _____ Duration _____minutes

Exercise _____ Duration _____minutes

Exercise _____ Duration _____minutes

Exercise _____ Duration _____minutes

■ **Record your brain-engaging activities for Week 7.**

_____

_____

_____

_____

■ **Record your stress-reducing activities for Week 7.**

_____

_____

_____

_____

■ **Record new ideas for brain-healthy meals and/or snacks that you plan to prepare or have already prepared.**

Breakfast _____

Lunch _____

Dinner _____

Snacks _____

■ **Record your weight at Week 7: _____**

WEEK 8 OF THE APT DIET

In Week 8, you will continue adjusting your diet to make it more brain-healthy (as detailed on page 144) and will also track your carbs, just as you did during Week 7. For the best results, note your exercise sessions, brain-engaging activities, and stress-reducing activities, as well as any new ideas you have for snacks and meals.

■ **Each day of Week 8, write down the foods you eat along with their carbohydrate counts. This will allow you to track your carbs throughout the day so that you can to stick to your Week 8 limit of 110 to 120 grams. At the end of each day, record your carb total.**

SUNDAY

Food _____ Carb grams _____

Food _____ Carb grams _____

Food _____ Carb grams _____

Food _____ Carb grams _____

Food _____ Carb grams _____

Food _____ Carb grams _____

Food _____ Carb grams _____

Food _____ Carb grams _____

Food _____ Carb grams _____

Food _____ Carb grams _____

Food _____ Carb grams _____

Food _____ Carb grams _____

Total carbs _____

MONDAY

Food _____ Carb grams _____

Food _____ Carb grams _____

Food _____ Carb grams _____

Food _____ Carb grams _____

Food _____ Carb grams _____

Food _____ Carb grams _____

Food _____ Carb grams _____

Food _____ Carb grams _____

Food _____ Carb grams _____

Food _____ Carb grams _____

Total carbs _____

TUESDAY

Food _____ Carb grams _____

Food _____ Carb grams _____

Food _____ Carb grams _____

Food _____ Carb grams _____

Food _____ Carb grams _____

Food _____ Carb grams _____

Food _____ Carb grams _____

Food _____ Carb grams _____

Food _____ Carb grams _____

Food _____ Carb grams _____

Total carbs _____

WEDNESDAY

Food _____ Carb grams _____

Food _____ Carb grams _____

Food _____ Carb grams _____

Food _____ Carb grams _____

Food _____ Carb grams _____

Food _____ Carb grams _____

Food _____ Carb grams _____

Food _____ Carb grams _____

Food _____ Carb grams _____

Food _____ Carb grams _____

Total carbs _____

THURSDAY

Food _____ Carb grams _____

Food _____ Carb grams _____

Food _____ Carb grams _____

Food _____ Carb grams _____

Food _____ Carb grams _____

Food _____ Carb grams _____

Food _____ Carb grams _____

Food _____ Carb grams _____

Food _____ Carb grams _____

Food _____ Carb grams _____

Total carbs _____

FRIDAY

Food _____ Carb grams _____

Food _____ Carb grams _____

Food _____ Carb grams _____

Food _____ Carb grams _____

Food _____ Carb grams _____

Food _____ Carb grams _____

Food _____ Carb grams _____

Food _____ Carb grams _____

Food _____ Carb grams _____

Food _____ Carb grams _____

Total carbs _____

SATURDAY

Food _____ Carb grams _____

Food _____ Carb grams _____

Food _____ Carb grams _____

Food _____ Carb grams _____

Food _____ Carb grams _____

Food _____ Carb grams _____

Food _____ Carb grams _____

Food _____ Carb grams _____

Food _____ Carb grams _____

Food _____ Carb grams _____

Total carbs _____

■ **Record your exercise sessions for Week 8.**

Exercise _____ Duration _____minutes

Exercise _____ Duration _____minutes

Exercise _____ Duration _____minutes

Exercise _____ Duration _____minutes

Exercise _____ Duration _____minutes

■ **Record your brain-engaging activities for Week 8.**

_____

_____

_____

_____

_____

■ **Record your stress-reducing activities for Week 8.**

_____

_____

_____

_____

_____

■ **Record new ideas for brain-healthy meals and/or snacks that you plan to prepare or have already prepared.**

Breakfast _____

Lunch _____

Dinner _____

Snacks _____

WEEK 9 OF THE APT DIET

In Week 9, you will make the final adjustments to your APT Diet (as detailed on page 147). For the final time, you will track your carbs each day and total them at the end of the day. As in the previous weeks, you should note your exercise sessions, brain-engaging activities, and stress-reducing activities, as well as any new ideas you have for snacks and meals. We encourage you to also list the snacks and meals that you've found most enjoyable over the last few weeks so that you can turn to these lists for menu ideas as you continue to follow your brain-healthy diet.

■ **List your ten favorite snacks and your ten favorite meals eaten over the previous weeks of the APT Diet.**

FAVORITE SNACKS

1. _____
2. _____
3. _____
4. _____
5. _____
6. _____
7. _____
8. _____
9. _____
10. _____

FAVORITE MEALS

1. _____
2. _____

3. _____

4. _____

5. _____

6. _____

7. _____

8. _____

9. _____

10. _____

■ Each day of Week 9, write down the foods you eat along with their carbohydrate counts. This will allow you to track your carbs throughout the day so that you can to stick to your Week 9 limit of 100 to 120 grams. At the end of each day, record your carb total.

SUNDAY

Food _____ Carb grams _____

Food _____ Carb grams _____

Food _____ Carb grams _____

Food _____ Carb grams _____

Food _____ Carb grams _____

Food _____ Carb grams _____

Food _____ Carb grams _____

Food _____ Carb grams _____

Food _____ Carb grams _____

Food _____ Carb grams _____

Total carbs _____

MONDAY

Food _____ Carb grams _____

Food _____ Carb grams _____

Food _____ Carb grams _____

Food _____ Carb grams _____

Food _____ Carb grams _____

Food _____ Carb grams _____

Food _____ Carb grams _____

Food _____ Carb grams _____

Food _____ Carb grams _____

Food _____ Carb grams _____

Total carbs _____

TUESDAY

Food _____ Carb grams _____

Food _____ Carb grams _____

Food _____ Carb grams _____

Food _____ Carb grams _____

Food _____ Carb grams _____

Food _____ Carb grams _____

Food _____ Carb grams _____

Food _____ Carb grams _____

Food _____ Carb grams _____

Food _____ Carb grams _____

Total carbs _____

WEDNESDAY

Food _____ Carb grams _____

Food _____ Carb grams _____

Food _____ Carb grams _____

Food _____ Carb grams _____

Food _____ Carb grams _____

Food _____ Carb grams _____

Food _____ Carb grams _____

Food _____ Carb grams _____

Food _____ Carb grams _____

Food _____ Carb grams _____

Total carbs _____

THURSDAY

Food _____ Carb grams _____

Food _____ Carb grams _____

Food _____ Carb grams _____

Food _____ Carb grams _____

Food _____ Carb grams _____

Food _____ Carb grams _____

Food _____ Carb grams _____

Food _____ Carb grams _____

Food _____ Carb grams _____

Food _____ Carb grams _____

Total carbs _____

FRIDAY

Food _____ Carb grams _____

Food _____ Carb grams _____

Food _____ Carb grams _____

Food _____ Carb grams _____

Food _____ Carb grams _____

Food _____ Carb grams _____

Food _____ Carb grams _____

Food _____ Carb grams _____

Food _____ Carb grams _____

Food _____ Carb grams _____

Total carbs _____

SATURDAY

Food _____ Carb grams _____

Food _____ Carb grams _____

Food _____ Carb grams _____

Food _____ Carb grams _____

Food _____ Carb grams _____

Food _____ Carb grams _____

Food _____ Carb grams _____

Food _____ Carb grams _____

Food _____ Carb grams _____

Food _____ Carb grams _____

Total carbs _____

■ **Record your exercise sessions for Week 9.**

Exercise _____ Duration _____minutes

Exercise _____ Duration _____minutes

Exercise _____ Duration _____minutes

Exercise _____ Duration _____minutes

Exercise _____ Duration _____minutes

■ **Record your brain-engaging activities for Week 9.**

_____

_____

_____

_____

_____

■ **Record your stress-reducing activities for Week 9.**

_____

_____

_____

_____

_____

■ **Record new ideas for brain-healthy meals and/or snacks that you plan to prepare or have already prepared.**

Breakfast _____

Lunch _____

Dinner _____

Snacks _____

Bibliography

Annweiler, C, DJ Llewellyn, and O Beauchet. "Low serum vitamin D concentrations in Alzheimer's disease: a systematic review and meta-analysis." *J Alzheimers Dis.* 2013; 33(3): 659–674.

Apelt, J, G Mehlhorn, and R Schliebs. "Insulin-sensitive GLUT4 glucose transporters are colocalized with GLUT3-expressing cells and demonstrate a chemically distinct neuron-specific localization in rat brain." *J Neurosci Res.* Sep 1999; 57(5): 693–705.

Avena, NM, P Rada, and BG Hoebel. "Sugar and fat bingeing have notable differences in addictive-like behavior." *J Nutr.* Mar 2009; 139(3): 623–628.

Barrios, D, C Greer, RS Isaacson, and CN Ochner. "Evidence surrounding the relation between coffee and cognitive function." *J Food Nutrition.* 2014; 1(1): 002.

Bayer-Carter, JL, et al. "Diet intervention and cerebrospinal fluid biomarkers in amnestic mild cognitive impairment." *Arch Neurol.* Jun 2011; 68(6): 743–752.

Beck, ME. "Dinner preparation in the modern United States." *British Food Journal.* 2007; 109(7): 531–547.

Bherer, L, KI Erickson, and T Liu-Ambrose. "A review of the effects of physical activity and exercise on cognitive and brain functions in older adults." *J Aging Res.* 2013; 2013: 657508.

Buchman, AS, et al. "Total daily physical activity and the risk of AD and cognitive decline in older adults." *Neurology.* Apr 2012; 78(17): 1323–1329.

Cao, C, et al. "Caffeine suppresses amyloid-beta levels in plasma and brain of Alzheimer's disease transgenic mice." *J Alzheimers Dis.* 2009; 17(3): 681–697.

Cao, C, et al. "High blood caffeine levels in MCI linked to lack of progression to dementia." *J Alzheimers Dis.* 2012; 30(3): 559–572.

Chapman, MJ, et al. "Effect of high-dose pitavastatin on glucose homeostasis in patients at elevated risk of new-onset diabetes: insights from the CAPITAIN and PREVAIL-US studies." *Curr Med Res Opin.* May 2014; 30(5): 775–784.

Connelly, PJ, et al. "A randomised double-blind placebo-controlled trial of folic acid supplementation of cholinesterase inhibitors in Alzheimer's disease." *Int J Geriatr Psychiatry.* Feb 2008; 23(2): 155–160.

Cotman, CW, NC Berchtold, and LA Christie. "Exercise builds brain health: key roles of growth factor cascades and inflammation." *Trends Neurosci.* Sep 2007; 30(9): 464–472.

Cummings, JL, RS Isaacson, FA Schmitt, and DM Velting. "A practical algorithm for managing Alzheimer's disease: what, when, and why?" *Ann Clin Transl Neurol.* Mar 2015; 2(3): 307–323.

Davangere, D, et al. "Olfactory identification deficits predict the transition from MCI to AD in a multi-ethnic community sample." *Alzheimers Dement.* July 2014; 10(4): P803.

de Jager, CA, et al. "Cognitive and clinical outcomes of homocysteine-lowering B-vitamin treatment in mild cognitive impairment: a randomized controlled trial." *Int J Geriatr Psychiatry.* June 2012; 27(6): 592–600.

de Villers-Sidani, E, et al. "Recovery of functional and structural age-related changes in the rat primary auditory cortex with operant training." *Proc Natl Acad Sci U S A.* Aug 2010; 107(31): 13900–13905.

DeSalvo, KB, R Olson, and KO Casavale. "Dietary guidelines for Americans." *JAMA.* Feb 2016; 315(5): 457–458.

Desideri, G, et al. "Benefits in cognitive function, blood pressure, and insulin resistance through cocoa flavanol consumption in elderly subjects with mild cognitive impairment: the Cocoa, Cognition, and Aging (CoCoA) study." *Hypertension.* Sep 2012; 60(3): 794–801.

Deters, F, and MR Mehl. "Does posting Facebook status updates increase or decrease loneliness? An online social networking experiment." *Social Psychological and Personality Science.* Sep 2013; 4(5): 579–586.

Devore, EE, et al. "Dietary intakes of berries and flavonoids in relation to cognitive decline." *Annal Neurol.* July 2012; 72(1): 135–143.

Douaud, G, et al. "Preventing Alzheimer's disease-related gray matter atrophy by B-vitamin treatment." *Proc Natl Acad Sci U S A.* June 2013; 110(23): 9523–9528.

Erickson, KI, et al. "The brain-derived neurotrophic factor Val[66]Met polymorphism moderates an effect of physical activity on working memory performance." *Psychol Sci.* Sep 2013; 24(9): 1770–1779.

Erickson, KI, et al. "Exercise training increases size of hippocampus and improves memory." *PNAS.* Jan 2011; 108(7): 3017–3022.

Fahnestock, M, et al. "BDNF increases with behavioral enrichment and an antioxidant diet in the aged dog." *Neurobiol Aging.* Mar 2012; 33(3): 546–554.

Fishel, MA, et al. "Hyperinsulinemia provokes synchronous increases in central inflammation and beta-amyloid in normal adults." *Arch Neurol.* Oct 2005; 62(10): 1539–1544.

Freund-Levi, Y, et al. "Omega-3 fatty acid treatment in 174 patients with mild to moderate Alzheimer disease: OmegAD study: a randomized double-blind trial." *Arch Neurol.* Oct 2006; 63(10): 1402–1408.

Fritsch, T, et al. "Cognitive functioning in healthy aging: the role of reserve and lifestyle factors early in life." *Gerontologist.* June 2007; 47(3): 307–322.

Gardener, SL, SR Rainey-Smith, and RN Martins. "Diet and inflammation in Alzheimer's disease and related chronic diseases: a review." *J Alzheimers Dis.* Dec 2015; 50(2): 301–334.

Glazer, H, C Greer, D Barrios, C Ochner, J Galvin, and R Isaacson. "Evidence on diet modification for Alzheimer's disease and mild cognitive impairment." *Neurology.* Apr 2014; 82(10): P5.224.

Green, RC, et al. "Disclosure of APOE genotype for risk of Alzheimer's disease." *N Engl J Med.* July 2009; 361(3): 245–254.

Growdon, ME, et al. "Odor identification and Alzheimer disease biomarkers in clinically normal elderly."*Neurology.* May 2015; 84(21): 2153–2160.

Gruen, I, et al. "Determination of cocoa flavor in chocolate ice creams by descriptive sensory analysis and SPME-GC volatile analysis." *Abstr Pap Am Chem Soc.* 1999; 218: U51.

Gutierrez, J, and R Isaacson. "Prevention of Cognitive Decline." *Handbook on the Neuropsychology of Aging and Dementia.* Ed. Lisa D. Ravdin and Heather L. Katzen. Springer Science & Business Media, LLC, 2013. 167–192. Print.

Hanna-Pladdy, B, and B Gajewski. "Recent and past musical activity predicts cognitive aging variability: direct comparison with general lifestyle activities." *Front Hum Neurosci.* July 2012; 6:198.

Hanson, AJ, et al. "Effect of apolipoprotein E genotype and diet on apolipoprotein E lipidation and amyloid peptides: randomized clinical trial." *JAMA Neurol.* Aug 2013; 70(8): 972–980.

Head, D, et al. "Exercise engagement as a moderator of the effects of APOE genotype on amyloid deposition." *Arch Neurol.* May 2012; 69(5): 636–643.

Henderson, ST, et al. "Study of ketogenic agent AC-1202 in mild to moderate Alzheimer's disease: a randomized, double-blind, placebo-controlled, multi-center trial." *Nutr Metab.* Aug 2009; 6: 31.

Hites, R, et al. "Global assessment of organic contaminants in farmed salmon." *Science.* Jan 2004; 303(5655): 226–229.

Hye, A, et al. "Plasma proteins predict conversion to dementia from prodromal disease." *Alzheimers Dement.* Nov 2014; 10(6): 799–807.

Ifland, JR, et al. "Refined food addiction: a classic substance use disorder." *Med Hypotheses.* May 2009; 72(5): 518–526.

Isaacson, RS, N Haynes, A Seifan, D Larsen, S Christiansen, JC Berger, JE Safdieh, AM Lunde, A Luo, M Kramps, M McInnis, and CN Ochner. "Alzheimer's prevention education: if we build it, will they come?" *J Prev Alz Dis.* Sep 2014; 1(2): 91–98.

Isaacson, RS, RD Khan, and CN Ochner. "Alzheimer's diet modification: a web-based nutrition tracking system for patient management and outcomes research." *J Nutrition Health & Aging.* Nov 2012; 16(9).

Jernerén, F, et al. "Brain atrophy in cognitively impaired elderly: the importance of long-chain w-3 fatty acids and B vitamin status in a randomized controlled trial." *Am J Clin Nutr.* July 2015; 102(1): 215–221.

Kanai, R, et al. "Online social network size is reflected in human brain structure." *Proc Biol Sci.* Apr 2012; 279(1732): 1327–1334.

Kerbage, Charles, et al. "Detection of ligand bound to beta amyloid in the lenses of human eyes." *Alzheimers Dement.* July 2014; 10(4): P173.

Kim, SY, J Karlawish, and BE Berkman. "Ethics of genetic and biomarker test disclosures in neurodegenerative disease prevention trials." *Neurology.* Apr 2015; 84(14): 1488–1494.

Kivipelto, M, et al. "The Finnish Geriatric Intervention Study to Prevent Cognitive Impairment and Disability (FINGER): study design and progress." *Alzheimers Dement.* Nov 2013; 9(6): 657–665.

Kliegel, M, D Zimprich, and C Rott. "Life-long intellectual activities mediate the predictive effect of early education on cognitive impairment in centenarians: a retrospective study." *Aging Ment Health.* Sep 2004; 8(5): 430–437.

Kraus, N. "Biological impact of music and software-based auditory training." *J Commun Disord.* Nov–Dec 2012; 45(6): 403–410.

Krikorian, R, et al. "Dietary ketosis enhances memory in mild cognitive impairment." *Neurobiol Aging.* Feb 2012; 33(2): 425.e19–27.

Leckie, RL, et al. "Potential moderators of physical activity on brain health." *J Aging Res.* 2012; 2012:948981.

Littlejohns, TJ, et al. "Vitamin D and dementia." *J Prev Alz Dis.* 2016; 3(1): 43–52.

Martin, B, MP Mattson, and S Maudsley. "Caloric restriction and intermittent fasting: two potential diets for successful brain aging." *Ageing Res Rev.* Aug 2006; 5(3): 332–353.

Mattson, MP, et al. "Meal frequency and timing in health and disease." *Proc Natl Acad Sci U S A.* Nov 2014; 111(47): 16647–16653.

Milgram, NW, et al. "Learning ability in aged beagle dogs is preserved by behavioral enrichment and dietary fortification: a two-year longitudinal study." *Neurobiol Aging.* Jan 2005; 26(1): 77–90.

Morris, MC, et al. "Association of seafood consumption, brain mercury level, and APOE ?4 status with brain neuropathology in older adults." *JAMA.* Feb 2016; 315(5): 489–497.

Morris, MC, et al. "MIND diet associated with reduced incidence of Alzheimer's disease." *Alzheimers Dement.* Sep 2015; 11(9): 1007–1014.

Morris, MC, et al. "MIND diet slows cognitive decline with aging." *Alzheimers Dement.* Sep 2015; 11(9): 1015–1022.

Mosconi, L, and PF McHugh. "Let food be thy medicine: diet, nutrition, and biomarkers' risk of Alzheimer's disease." *Curr Nutr Rep.* June 2015; 4(2): 126–135.

Naderali, EK, SH Ratcliffe, and MC Dale. "Obesity and Alzheimer's disease: a link between body weight and cognitive function in old age." *Am J Alzheimers Dis Other Demen.* Dec 2009–Jan 2010; 24(6): 445–449.

Neafsey, EJ, and MA Collins. "Moderate alcohol consumption and cognitive risk." *Neuropsychiatr Dis Treat.* 2011; 7: 465–484.

Ngandu, T, et al. "A 2 year multidomain intervention of diet, exercise, cognitive training, and vascular risk monitoring versus control to prevent cognitive decline in at-risk elderly people (FINGER): a randomised controlled trial." *Lancet.* June 2015; 385(9984): 2255–2263.

Norton, S, et al. "Potential for primary prevention of Alzheimer's disease: an analysis of population-based data." *Lancet Neurology.* Aug 2014; 13(8): 788–794.

Oboudiyat, C, H Glazer, A Seifan, C Greer, and RS Isaacson. "Alzheimer's disease." *Semin Neurol.* Sep 2013; 33(4): 313–329.

Padilla, C, and R Isaacson. "Genetics of dementia." *Continuum*. Apr 2011; 17(2 Neurogenetics): 326–342.

Paganini-Hill, A, CH Kawas, and MM Corrada. "Lifestyle factors and dementia in the oldest-old: The 90+ Study." *Alzheimer Dis Assoc Disord*. Mar 2015.

Pasinetti, FM, et al. "Roles of resveratrol and other grape-derived polyphenols in Alzheimer's disease prevention and treatment." *Biochim Biophys Acta*. June 2015; 1852(6): 1202–1208.

Patterson, CE, SA Todd, and AP Passmore. "Effect of apolipoprotein E and butyrylcholinesterase genotypes on cognitive response to cholinesterase inhibitor treatment at different stages of Alzheimer's disease." *Pharmacogenomics J*. Dec 2011; 11(6): 444–450.

Pop, V, et al. "Synergistic effects of long-term antioxidant diet and behavioral enrichment on beta-amyloid load and non-amyloidogenic processing in aged canines." *J Neurosci*. July 2010; 30(29): 9831–9839.

Quinn, JF, et al. "A clinical trial of docosahexanoic acid (DHA) for the treatment of Alzheimer's disease." *Alzheimers Dement*. July 2009; 5(4): P84.

Quinn, JF, et al. "Docosahexaenoic acid supplementation and cognitive decline in Alzheimer disease: a randomized trial." *JAMA*. Nov 2010; 304(17): 1903–1911.

Rada, P, NM Avena, and BG Hoebel. "Daily bingeing on sugar repeatedly releases dopamine in the accumbens shell." *Neuroscience*. 2005; 134(3): 737–744.

Read, S, P Wu, and M Biscow. "Sustained 4-year cognitive and functional response in early Alzheimer's disease with pioglitazone." *J Am Geriatr Soc*. Mar 2014; 62(3): 584–586.

Reas, ET, et al. "Moderate, regular alcohol consumption is associated with higher cognitive function in older community-dwelling adults." *J Prev Alz Dis*. 2016; 3(1).

Reed, BR, et al. "Cognitive activities during adulthood are more important than education in building reserve." *J Int Neuropsychol Soc*. July 2011; 17(4): 615–624.

Reger, MA, et al. "Effects of beta-hydroxybutyrate on cognition in memory-impaired adults." *Neurobiol Aging*. Mar 2004; 25(3): 311–314.

Richardson, JR, et al. "Elevated serum pesticide levels and risk for Alzheimer disease." *JAMA Neurol*. Mar 2014; 71(3): 284–290.

Ringman, JM, et al. "Oral curcumin for Alzheimer's disease: tolerability and efficacy in a 24-week randomized, double blind, placebo-controlled study." *Alzheimers Res Ther*. Oct 2012; 4(5): 43.

Roberts, RO, et al. "Relative intake of macronutrients impacts risk of mild cognitive impairment or dementia." *J Alzheimers Dis*. Jan 2012; 32(2): 329–339.

Rouch, L, et al. "Antihypertensive drugs, prevention of cognitive decline and dementia: a systematic review of observational studies, randomized controlled trials and meta-analyses, with discussion of potential mechanisms." *CNS Drugs.* Feb 2015; 29(2): 113–130.

Särkämö, T, et al. "Cognitive, emotional, and social benefits of regular musical activities in early dementia: randomized controlled study." *Gerontologist.* Aug 2014; 54(4): 634–650.

Satizabal, CL, et al. "Temporal trends in dementia incidence in the Framingham study." *Alzheimers Dement.* July 2014; 10(4): P296.

Scarmeas, N, et al. "Mediterranean diet and mild cognitive impairment." *Arch Neurol.* Feb 2009; 66(2): 216–225.

Seifan, A, and RS Isaacson. "The Alzheimer's Prevention Clinic at Weill Cornell Medicince and NewYork-Presbyterian: risk stratification and personalized early intervention." *J Prev Alz Dis.* Oct 2015; 2(4): 254–266.

Smith, AD, and K Yaffe. "Dementia (including Alzheimer's disease) can be prevented: statement supported by international experts." *J Alzheimers Dis.* 2014; 38(4): 699–703.

Smith, AD, et al. "Homocysteine-lowering by B vitamins slows the rate of accelerated brain atrophy in mild cognitive impairment: a randomized controlled trial." *PLoS One.* Sep 2010; 5(9): e12244.

Smith, JC, et al. "Physical activity reduces hippocampal atrophy in elders at genetic risk for Alzheimer's disease." *Front Aging Neurosci.* 2014; 6: 61.

Smith, PJ, and JA Blumenthal. "Dietary factors and cognitive decline." *J Prev Alz Dis.* 2016; 3(1): 53–64.

Sparks, DL, et al. "Circulating cholesterol levels, apolipoprotein E genotype and dementia severity influence the benefit of atorvastatin treatment in Alzheimer's disease: results of the Alzheimer's Disease Cholesterol-Lowering Treatment (ADCLT) trial." *Acta Neurol Scand Suppl.* 2006; 185: 3–7.

Sperling, R, E Mormino, and K Johnson. "The evolution of preclinical Alzheimer's disease: implications for prevention trials." *Neuron.* Nov 2014; 84(3): 608–622.

Sperling, RA, et al. "Toward defining the preclinical stages of Alzheimer's disease: recommendations from the National Institute on Aging-Alzheimer's Association workgroups on diagnostic guidelines for Alzheimer's disease." *Alzheimers Dement.* May 2011; 7(3): 280–292.

US Department of Health and Human Services. "2015–2020 Dietary Guidelines for Americans, 8th edition." Office of Disease Prevention and Health Promotion. Dec 2015. www.health.gov/DietaryGuidelines/2015/Guidelines.

Vellas, B, et al. "Long-term use of standardised Ginkgo biloba extract for the prevention of Alzheimer's disease (GuidAge): a randomised placebo-controlled trial." *Lancet Neurol.* Oct 2012; 11(10): 851–859.

Vellas, B, et al. "MAPT (multi-domain Alzheimer's prevention trial): clinical, biomarkers results and lessons for the future." *J Prev Alz Dis.* 2015; 2(4) 292–293.

Wang, J, et al. "Cocoa extracts reduce oligomerization of amyloid-β: implications for cognitive improvement in Alzheimer's disease." *J Alzheimers Dis.* 2014; 41(2): 643–650.

Wells, RE, et al. "Meditation's impact on default mode network and hippocampus in mild cognitive impairment: a pilot study." *Neurosci Lett.* Nov 2013; 27(556): 15–19.

Whitmer, RA, et al. "Central obesity and increased risk of dementia more than three decades later." *Neurology.* Sep 2008; 71(14): 1057–1064.

Williams, JW, et al. "Preventing Alzheimer's disease and cognitive decline." *Evidence Reports/Technology Assessments.* Apr 2010; 193: 1–727.

Witte, AV, et al. "Effects of resveratrol on memory performance, hippocampal functional connectivity, and glucose metabolism in healthy older adults." *J Neurosci.* June 2014; 34(23): 7862–7870.

World Health Organization. "Q&A on the carcinogenicity of the consumption of red meat and processed meat." Online Q&A. October 2015.

Yurko-Mauro, K, et al. "Beneficial effects of docosahexaenoic acid on cognition in age-related cognitive decline." *Alzheimers Dement.* Nov 2010; 6(6): 456–464.

About the Authors

Richard S. Isaacson, MD, received his bachelor's and medical degrees from the University of Missouri—Kansas City School of Medicine. He completed his residency in Neurology at Beth Israel Deaconess Medical Center/Harvard Medical School, and his medical internship at Mount Sinai Medical Center in Miami Beach, Florida.

Dr. Isaacson has served as Associate Medical Director of the Wien Center for Alzheimer's Disease and Memory Disorders at Mount Sinai Medical Center in Florida; and as Associate Professor of Clinical Neurology, Vice Chair of Education, and Education Director of the McKnight Brain Institute in the Department of Neurology at the University of Miami Miller School of Medicine. He is the founder and the director of the Alzheimer's Prevention Clinic at Weill Cornell Medicine and New York-Presbyterian, where he presently serves as Associate Professor of Neurology and Director of the Neurology Residency Training Program.

Dr. Isaacson specializes exclusively in Alzheimer's disease risk reduction and treatment, mild cognitive impairment due to AD, and pre-clinical AD. His research focuses on nutrition and the implementation and assessment of dietary interventions for AD management. The doctor's recent efforts have focused on the development of Alzheimer's Universe (www.AlzU.org), a vast online educational portal on AD prevention and treatment available to the public. AlzU.org has been shown to significantly improve knowledge about AD with results published in the *Journal of Prevention of Alzheimer's Disease,* and has reached over 150,000 people in thirty-six countries. Dr. Isaacson is also the author of *Alzheimer's Treatment Alzheimer's Prevention: A Patient and Family Guide.*

Christopher N. Ochner, PhD, completed two master's degrees in Psychology and a master's in Biostatistics at Columbia University in New York, and received his PhD in Clinical Psychology at Drexel University in Philadelphia. He then completed an individual NIH grant fellowship at the Columbia University Institute of Human Nutrition/New York Obesity Nutrition Research Center, managing the center's largest clinical research laboratory.

In 2009, Dr. Ochner received an NIH career development award and was promoted to the faculty of the Columbia University College of Physicians and Surgeons. He became the youngest Columbia faculty to form and run an independent research laboratory, publishing a number of peer-reviewed articles related to nutrition. He was then recruited to the Icahn School of Medicine at Mount Sinai as the Director of Research Development and Administration to establish and direct a portfolio of clinical research studies based on nutrition. He is now President and CEO of The Nutrition Science Initiative (NuSI), a nonprofit organization that facilitates and funds experimental research in nutrition.

Dr. Ochner is an internationally known nutrition expert, lecturing around the world and appearing widely in the media, including *The New York Times, The Wall Street Journal, USA Today,* and *Good Morning America.* He also serves as Editor-in-Chief for the *International Journal of Nutrition* and is an International Advisory Board Member for *The Lancet Diabetes & Endocrinology.*

$\mathscr{I}$ndex

GLYCEMIC INDEX FOOD GUIDE

For Weight Loss, Cardiovascular Health, Diabetic Management, and Maximum Energy

Dr. Shari Lieberman

The glycemic index (GI) is an important nutritional tool. By indicating how quickly a given food triggers a rise in blood sugar, the GI enables you to choose foods that can help you manage a variety of conditions, as well as improve your overall health.

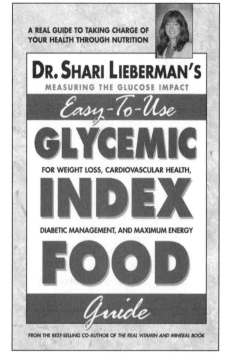

Written by Dr. Shari Lieberman, one of America's leading nutritionists, this book was designed as an easy-to-use guide to the glycemic index. The book first looks at commonly asked questions about the GI. What are carbohydrates, and what do they have to do with the GI? How is the GI of a food calculated? What is glycemic load? How are high-GI foods associated with diabetes, obesity, and other health problems? How can a low-GI diet improve your health? The author answers these questions and more, ensuring that you truly understand the index and know how to use it. She then provides both the glycemic index and the glycemic load of hundreds of foods and beverages, including raw foods, cooked foods, and many combination and prepared foods. Throughout, helpful tips guide you towards the best dietary choices.

Whether you are interested in controlling your glucose levels to manage your diabetes, lose weight, increase your heart health, boost your energy level, or simply enhance your well-being, the *Glycemic Index Food Guide* is the best place to start.

$7.95 US • 160 pages • 4 x 7-inch mass paperback • ISBN 978-0-7570-0245-8

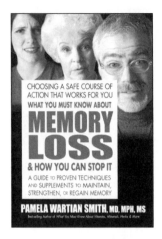

WHAT YOU MUST KNOW ABOUT MEMORY LOSS & HOW YOU CAN STOP IT

A Guide to Proven Techniques and Supplements to Maintain, Strengthen, or Regain Memory

Pamela Wartian Smith, MD, MPH, MS

With over 77 million baby boomers living in the U.S., memory loss is fast becoming a major issue. Although the common belief is that these lapses are a normal part of aging, research indicates that there are a number of reasons they can occur. In *What You Must Know About Memory Loss & How You Can Stop It,* Dr. Pamela Wartian Smith looks at the possible causes and explains what you can do to not only reverse the problem but also enhance your ability to focus on, comprehend, and recall information.

If you or a loved one is troubled by memory loss, or if you want to optimize both your memory and your overall brain function, Dr. Smith provides simple and effective solutions.

$15.95 US • 240 pages • 6 x 9-inch quality paperback • ISBN 978-0-7570-0386-8

SOFT FOODS FOR EASIER EATING COOKBOOK

Easy-to-Follow Recipes for People Who Have Chewing and Swallowing Problems

Sandra Woodruff, RD, and Leah Gilbert-Henderson, PhD

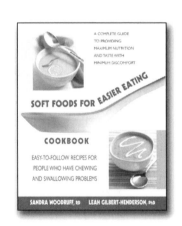

Each year, medical treatments leave millions of patients with chewing and swallowing difficulties. While most hospitals deal with this by puréeing their food, the results are unappetizing. To solve this problem, Sandra Woodruff and Leah Gilbert-Henderson have written *Soft Foods for Easier Eating Cookbook,* an easy-to-follow guide that offers maximum nutrition and taste with minimum discomfort. After presenting simple strategies for living with chewing and swallowing difficulties, the authors provide over 150 recipes for smashing smoothies, sumptuous soups, hearty entrées, and much more.

$18.95 US • 320 pages • 7.5 x 9-inch quality paperback • ISBN 978-0-7570-0290-8

Overcoming Senior Moments
Vanishing Thoughts—Causes and Remedies
Frances Meiser and Nina Anderson

Millions of Americans suffer from Alzheimer's disease, and each year, a greater number of young people are diagnosed with this devastating illness. In *Overcoming Senior Moments,* Frances Meiser and Nina Anderson provide simple but effective techniques to advance brain function and prevent memory loss in people of all ages.

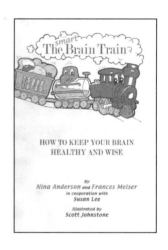

The book begins with an explanation of memory loss and its basic remedies. Using direct language and clear illustrations, the authors explore ways to maintain brain health, guard against dementia, and improve cognition. Also included is a list of recommended supplements and a directory of resources.

$9.95 US • 88 pages • 6 x 9-inch quality paperback • ISBN 978-0-9701110-9-8

The Smart Brain Train
How to Keep Your Brain Healthy and Wise
Nina Anderson and Frances Meiser
Illustrated by Scott Johnstone

This delightful book offers a nutritional approach to improving children's brain health. The authors first address the child, explaining the importance of water, exercise, and diet in brain development. They then offer vital supplemental information for parents, who are encouraged to take an active role in their child's development. A progress chart, to be filled in by parents and kids together, makes it easy to improve dietary habits.

With the right nutrition and their parents' help, children can achieve higher levels of learning. *The Smart Brain Train* helps families work together toward this important goal.

$7.95 US • 56 pages • 6 x 9-inch quality paperback • ISBN 978-1-884820-87-8

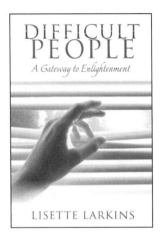

DIFFICULT PEOPLE
A Gateway to Enlightenment
Lisette Larkins

For most of us, difficult people (DPs) are the bane of our existence. But it is also true that DPs mirror our own dysfunctional mental states and provide us with wonderful opportunities to understand and heal ourselves.

Lisette Larkins realized the positive aspect of dealing with difficult people when she was providing care for a late-stage Alzheimer's patient. This began a personal journey of exploration that ultimately led to Larkins' spiritual awakening. In *Difficult People: A Gateway to Enlightenment,* she shares her journey and guides readers in reaching a "chronic state of well-being."

$17.95 US • 256 pages • 5.5 x 8.5-inch quality paperback • ISBN 978-0-9844955-6-6

BLUE SKY, WHITE CLOUDS
A Book for Memory-Challenged Adults
Eliezer Sobel

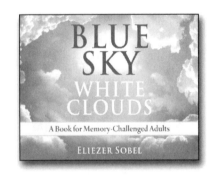

In working with his eighty-six-year-old mother, who was in the advanced stages of Alzheimer's disease, author Eliezer Sobel made an astounding discovery. Although she could not speak full sentences or follow a story line, his mother could still read, and would sit in rapt attention as she paged through magazines and coffee-table books. To accommodate and encourage his mother's love of reading, Sobel wrote *Blue Sky, White Clouds.* A simple picture book with beautiful photographs and large, easy-to-read type, this is a perfect gift for any loved one who has Alzheimer's disease or dementia.

$19.95 US • 36 pages • 11 x 8.5-inch hardback • ISBN 978-1-937907-07-5